THE
ORIGINAL BODY

Primal Movement for Yoga Teachers

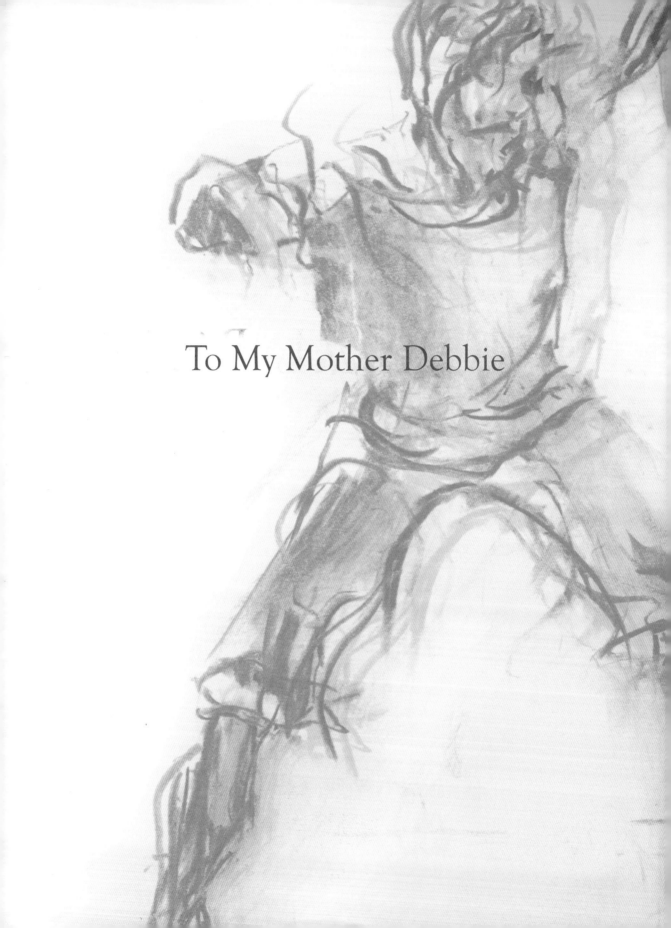

To My Mother Debbie

THE
ORIGINAL BODY

Primal Movement for Yoga Teachers

John Stirk

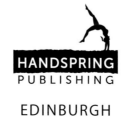

HANDSPRING
PUBLISHING

EDINBURGH

HANDSPRING PUBLISHING LIMITED
The Old Manse, Fountainhall,
Pencaitland, East Lothian
EH34 5EY, United Kingdom
Tel: +44 1875 341 859
Website: www.handspringpublishing.com

First published 2015 in the United Kingdom by Handspring Publishing
Reprinted 2016

ISBN 978-1-909141-25-4

British Library Cataloguing in Publication Data
A catalogue record for this book is available from the British Library

Important notice
Neither the publishers nor the authors will be liable for any loss or damage of any nature occasioned
to or suffered by any person or property in regard to product liability, negligence or otherwise, or through acting
or refraining from acting as a result of adherence to the material contained in this book.

Commissioning Editor Sarena Wolfaard, Handspring Publishing Limited
Design direction and illustration by Bruce Hogarth, kinesis-creative
Cover design by Bruce Hogarth, kinesis-creative
Cover illustration by Lisa Joffe
Copy editing by Lee Bowers
Typeset by DiTech Process Solutions
Printed by Pulsio, Sofia, Bulgaria
Index by DiTech Process Solutions

Contents

Comments from Students and Teachers

"Over the past nearly 20 years, my work with John has been by far the biggest influence on my teaching and success with my students. I have had the privilege to take workshops and experience many excellent yoga teachers and John's work continues to be the deepest, most powerful, and is always new. John's knowledge of the body and the *work* enables me to communicate with my students on how they too can deeply relate and connect yoga to their own bodies - a gift that they use to deepen their practice. From my students that are themselves also teachers, I hear: 'Wow, I have been practicing for years, but this is the first time I have noticed...We should all be teaching this way!'"

Trish Strauss - Breath and Balance Yoga Studio, New Hampshire, USA.

"I have been a student of John's for over 25 years and I am still enthralled by his ongoing development and depth of knowledge. His unique style of teaching combines a deep understanding of yoga and wealth of experience as an osteopath, the results being much more than the sum of two parts. Each class is a journey of discovery, engaging with the inherent intelligence of the body and encouraging its powers of self-healing."

Nadine Hobson - Osteopath, UK.

"Working with John brings focus to my movement, my breath unravels with a sense of purpose and my spine flows into richer movement from a much deeper connection."

Ana Barretxeguren - Pilates teacher and Myofascial Release practitioner, UK.

"As a teacher training young actors and dancers I have found John's work invaluable in providing a unique insight into the inner mechanisms of the body supporting both vocal and physical development. The work is an original and detailed biomechanical approach to the human organism, it is inherently inclusive, everyone is able to do the simple positions. An essential tool for anyone involved in movement training."

Rose Ryan - Lecturer in Theatre and Dance, UK.

"This work is like giving oneself a very deeply personal treatment/session that is enhanced because I am doing it to myself and so have the complete responsibility for accessing whatever part of me, and however deeply I want to take it, rather than seeking this from an outside source (another practitioner)."

Jo Brook - Zero Balancing practitioner, UK.

"John's work has enabled me to gain knowledge of the highest level about the workings of my body and my mind (the body brain). If you were born with a constant hunger to express and explore the physical self (as I was), you will never be satisfied with a method. His way of working, which is not only creative, unique, challenging and healing, is also richly infused with anatomical detail, allowing me to access the deepest tissue layers of my body and thus metamorphose into a more fearless dancing creature."

Megan Schirra - creative body worker, dancer, Switzerland.

Foreword

There are many people that think that everyone we meet can change our lives, a theory that I ascribe to, with the rider that some have the ability to change us more than others, and John Stirk definitely falls into that category, in spades.

I was fortunate enough to meet John in 1985, when, of course, everything was in black and white, and he was my first hatha yoga teacher, teaching me weekly, one-on-ones for about a year in a wooden floored room above a trendy restaurant in Maida Vale, and then a weekly small group of my friends in my house. Through the practice that John taught, the way I lived my life, as they say in marketing, took a strong upward curve, and quite a few years late I gave up practising law and eventually launched Tri-yoga. His teaching then, as it is now, was original, authentic and unique.

Over the years, it has been my honour to either practice under or work alongside some amazing yoga teachers as they teach from Tri-yoga. And I am often asked what we look for in a teacher, which is a mixture of attributes. There is a blend of sound and deep knowledge, safety, the ability to communicate, teaching from their own experience, a genuine sense of care for their students, and ultimately the ability to inspire others to have their own practice.

And there's a bit more: yoga is a practice of growth and courage; it's not about being satisfied where we've got to. Inspiring teachers continue to extend and deepen their practice and out of their generosity pass their experience on to us so that we may take ourselves where we need to go.

From my first experiences of being taught by John to today, he does all of that, and with his own twist, his own humour, his own warmth and his soft yet consistent drive for our growth. His teaching is never stationery; every class or workshop is different and brings something new. Yet you know, even if you feel almost uncertain, at the same time you know that you are in safe hands. And his teaching has an openness, an awareness that there is no one way of being in a pose that we all have to fit to, whatever the shape or formation of our individual bodies – this in turn allows us to have our own practice for our own body.

His teaching and this book reflect his perpetual thirst to deepen and expand himself, and share from his own experience in both stillness to movement so we can look after our own original bodies.

The Original Body is a guide from someone who has been involved in teaching the practice of yoga for over forty years and feels almost commanded to ensure that the real essence of yoga, the 'necessity' to turn within, is not lost in the West. It's a guide for teachers and students and anyone with an interest. It feels like the guide shows us, and the reader chooses, the how and maybe the why.

All of this means that John's students can come from the most experienced teachers who regularly go to his classes and workshops to beginners who will have found a great way to start their yoga practice.

I know without doubt I would not be where I am today if I hadn't had the good fortune to have been taught by John.

Jonathan Sattin
Founder and Managing Director Triyoga, London UK
2015

Acknowledgements

I would like to thank the many students over the years, who have made a significant contribution to this book, particularly my co-explorers for their continued interest, curiosity, receptivity, trust, and their willingness to move in new directions.

I would like to thank Howard Evans for his faith and advice in this project, Graham Tomlin for his patience and guidance in computer skills, Sarah Stirk for her artistic eye and photography, Lolly Stirk for her constant faith in me and for her ideas, Lisa Joffe, Bruce Hogarth and Nicola Fee for their artwork and Sarena Wolfaard at Handspring Publishers for her level of engagement. I would also like to thank my London students who agreed to have their images in this book.

I would also like to mention some of the pioneers, who have helped further the evolution of body and mind work, and have been particularly influential in supporting my own inquiry. I am particularly grateful to BKS Iyengar and Vanda Scaravelli, for their inspired and innovative practice and teaching, John Wernham for sustaining the light and scope of classical osteopathy , Ida Rolf for highlighting the relevance of connective tissue, Moshe Feldenkrais for his investigations into awareness through movement, Emilie Conrad for her ground breaking work with the fluid body, and R.D. Laing and J. Krishnamurti, who in their direct and sensitive way, drew attention to 'how we are' in relationship, with ourselves and with others. I continue to be indebted to the concept of yoga and those who pioneered its inception.

Introduction

This book highlights the deeper experience of the teacher as the essential aspect in guiding, and inspiring others. *The Original Body* supports personal inquiry, and, while steering away from methods, recognises the need for a working framework. The intention of this book is to draw out a deeper experience by enhancing the ability to 'go in to oneself' and to use this as a primary foundation for teaching. A deeper practice deepens *us* and our skills.

A personal experiment, such as yoga, is original for each of us. We start with our self, within or without a group. Originality implies an unknown element and suggests that everything we know about ourselves is organised around an original body, a primal nature submerged beneath a layer of conditioning, including, on occasion, the conditioning of yoga itself.

Yoga postures are not always the best mechanical option for change and there is much debate concerning how they should be performed, if performance is the right word. If we let go of an emphasis on range of movement and set positions, things begin to look simpler, refreshingly creative and have the potential for a deeper experience.

Goethe said, 'If you cannot find words to describe it you are on the right path.' Einstein commented, 'The most beautiful thing we can experience is the mysterious, it is the source of all true art and science.' Krishnamurti taught that releasing ourselves from the grip of 'what we know gives a sense of boundless freedom'. If life had no mystery there would be few life sciences and no *unknown* to surrender to. This book highlights exploration as a route to a more profound experience while acknowledging an unobtainable factor as an element of our discoveries.

There are some aspects of our evolutionary journey that may never be known. It is accepted that ultimately we evolved in an aquatic environment eons ago, and that the neocortex is a relatively new development. Add to this the realisation that for the majority the body-mind could benefit from some work and that the cortex and its ideas might learn from its prehistory, and you have the basis for an approach founded on millions of years of physiological experience.

There is a way of moving that harks back to a time before yoga was thought of, before thought itself. There are ways of being moved that feel so ancient that they are best understood as underpinning all other movements and positons. We have a personal and a common originality. We are individuals springing from a common base. When personal patterns are pared back we tend to exhibit the same behaviour.

The term 'Original' refers to the authentic inquiry of each practitioner, recognises each practitioner as an individual, and also refers to the ancient properties of the organism. An original practice reveals an original body. We move in a primordial way as a consequence of moving into and through ourselves. The fact that we are individually original is reflected in speech, thought, walking, ways of being and personal behaviour. We also originate from the same source, the same evolutionary roots. As we have moved up the evolutionary ladder the more individual we have become. Our highly developed nervous system provides an acute awareness that 'we are', rendering us more susceptible to external influence, to each other, and to our own sensitivity.

When we pass through personal patterning, an original body emerges that dissolves individual differences. *We begin to move in the same way.* Regardless of positional constructs, or styles of movement, we become aware of our common originality. Primal movement predates yoga, draws on a deeper activity residing beneath conditioning and arises as an individual discovery. The spontaneous behaviour of the organism and the adjustments needed to enable its emergence are moment-to-moment aspects of the same process. Conscious awareness and the natural expression of the body feed each other as voluntary and involuntary movement conspire to produce an enriching and enlightening practice.

Science has studied energy, consciousness, love and yoga, but it still seeks a connection between the chemistry of experience and actual experience. While science continues to explore the factors that make us tick, we continue to explore ourselves, and as our experience deepens we come to our own conclusions. Science may support our experience to a point but cannot provide the experience of being 'in it'. All experience is physiological. You cannot change physiology without changing yourself.

There is no ideal state. Relaxation might come close to an ideal, but we have not evolved through relaxation. We have had to work for relaxation. We have birthed ourselves and applied effort to counter the stresses of life. There are, however, 'preferable states' that might include a body free from pain and impediments, that moves with ease and grace, a body we gain pleasure from, and a mind that is at least relatively free from the grip of non-essential repetitive thought, a mind less controlled by itself.

Experience shows that deeper work has the potential for ever deepening and ever changing. We cannot 'know' it. Physiology reveals itself in its own unique way. Primal movement has no agenda other than to express itself, and it does so simply because it can. Origination reveals itself by removing everything in its wake; it wipes the slate clean, at least for the time being.

The only way I have been able to write this book is by letting go to it, by writing it in a way that exemplifies its message, that is by sinking beneath the information supporting it and practising what I preach in the writing. The paradox is that the more information I discovered the more I became seduced by the feeling that the organism knows so much more once we learn to yield ourselves to it. Word language is limited in its ability to convey the scope of sensory appreciation, but remains one of the few effective tools of communication available.

I have strayed from traditional frameworks while continuing to represent what is, in my opinion the essence of yoga. Western and Eastern principles and practices recognise our individuality in relation to a bigger picture, and that change takes work. *The Original Body* is the culmination of 40 years of personal inquiry into the experiential field of the body-mind. The main input has been primarily provided by the practice of yoga and osteopathy but includes exposure to a range of body and mind disciplines. The insights arising from their combination have been personally profound and invaluable in guiding others towards a similar experience. All experience is physiological. You cannot change physiology without changing yourself. Physical changes provide a springboard for a more complete experience and outcome. While the references herein apply to inspiring individuals that have made a significant contribution to a faith in my own experience and a trust in my perceptions, this book remains a consequence of work on myself, by myself, and its aim is to encourage others to trust in their own process.

Who This Book is for and How to Use It

This book is for yoga teachers and students interested in deepening their experience and understanding, but may also interest those practicing and teaching other body-mind activities. This book can be used as a springboard for taking you further into yourself for inspiring teaching.

You can use this book as a door to pass through, and pass through again, until practice transforms into an experience beyond methods and ideas surrounding practice. Use this book to cultivate a deeper feeling in your body, to sense between your vertebrae, to discover the potential depth of your articulations and the extent of your inner space and fluidity.

The exercises can be used to underpin ongoing positional work or as a practice. The practical application of 'deep work' may be sufficient and take the place of, or run parallel to, existing practices.

I have been particularly selective with the anatomical and biomechanical aspects to maintain a simple and direct approach. Experience shows that too much detail clutters awareness as opposed to enhancing it. The anatomical figures relate primarily to skeletal aspects because of the clarity afforded by their visualization and the important role they play in our sensory imagination. 'The work' brings articulation into focus. The bones and the spaces between them form a reliable ongoing guide leading to a deeper sensory experience on other levels. Helpful material on anatomy and yoga can be found elsewhere. Primal movement, like all movement, is realised through feeling. *Feeling deeper movement provides a deeper understanding.* You can visualise the anatomical aspects of this book as a sensory guide to confirm what you feel and where you feel it. There comes a point when all information, as useful as it is, is dissolved by the depth of practice. Everything that has been said and understood on the subject evaporates into pure in-the-moment experience. This book provides a stepping stone.

This book focuses on physical exploration but also returns to what may be seen as familiar ground on other levels. The question of 'how we are' is fundamental to all body-mind work. Practice begins with what we do and becomes what we are. Doing and being are two sides of the same coin. Yoga lies beneath all patterns of human conditioning while originality lies beneath all forms of yoga. The yoga masters understood that a framework is needed as a door to the yoga experience and beyond, and that the door itself was not it. Deepening physiological awakening deepens awakening on all levels. New discoveries continue to enrich practice and teaching. This book can be used for taking you and others with you, into a rich and enlightening experience.

People come to yoga expecting change. They are usually not disappointed. A potential for change exists that arises from a depth within the organism, the intensity of which is unexpected. There are places within us and ways of moving that lie dormant. When awakened, they provide the deep transformation that yoga offers.

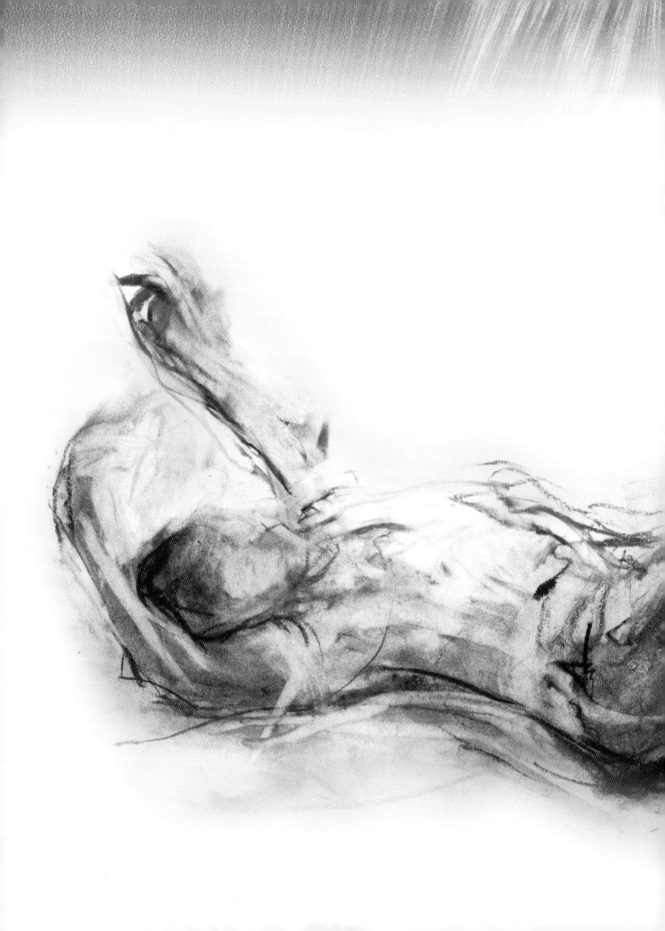

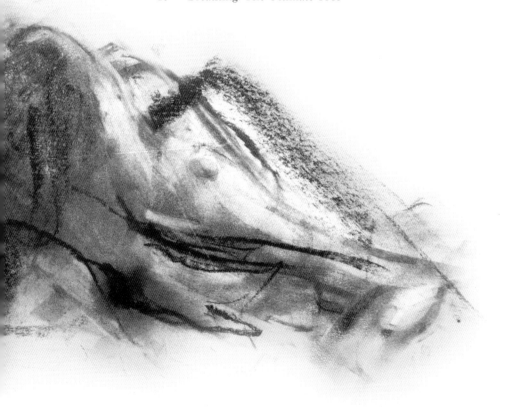

The Original Body

Something Within

There is something deeply within us, a movement, a rhythm, an energy that through lack of acknowledgement and habitual conditioning lies dormant. Its elusiveness may prevail in spite of yoga practice but it awakens when conditions are favourable. The awakening is initially physiological but then spreads into other areas of our experience.

All movement is an expression of life. Heartbeat, peristalsis and other organic rhythms are considered involuntary and more or less beyond the control of volition, while the movements we *use* in life are voluntary. Life's essential experiences are also involuntary. Childbirth and orgasm are prime examples of involuntary forces at work. Physiology, if encouraged, takes over. We are taken by the body, and surrender to its process.

There is an involuntary potential within us that seeks powerful expression. It is physiologically potent, intelligently mobile, its release affects us on all levels, and it surfaces in the absence of volitional control. We may be familiar with the spontaneous elongation of the spine, yet a potential exists for the emergence of an activity that is particularly deep and strong. It spreads throughout the entire system, places the feet firmly on the ground, activates the soft tissues and opens the articulations. Primal movement reveals an intelligence and strength that goes beyond spinal elongation. It releases an activity that lies beneath personal patterns, methods or ideas about what we should or should not be doing.

Involuntary movement of this kind has expressed, or attempted to express itself, long before the advent of yoga and similar activities, long before body-mind work of any kind was thought of, before thought itself. We can bring this movement to life. We can realise a skeletal, soft tissue, articular and fluid way of moving that underpins, informs and enhances all postures. Retrieving involuntary action involves deep inquiry, but then we can allow it to happen. Primal movement provides an original experience during active or restful practice.

Self-Evidence

Scientific inquiry confirms that yoga works. Science became interested in yoga because of individual experience. The apparent beneficial effects to yoga practitioners triggered studies highlighting the value of traditional practices. Positive physiological responses to hatha yoga and meditation practice have been well documented (Funderburk 1977). Research is ongoing, and evidence-based research has led to yoga's inclusion in school curricula, hospitals, and a variety of institutions and associations concerned with the health and well-being of their members and students. The current global attraction to yoga has been stimulated for various reasons. Yoga feels good, has the potential for changing how we are on several levels, and has a spiritual dimension. Whether practised in groups or alone, yoga involves each practitioner 'going inwards' and doing the work. For many centuries yoga's efficacy has been self-evident. The effectiveness of yoga as an experiential science is self-evident to those of us who practice it. Scientific confirmation of its efficacy is supportive. But discoveries arise because we go inwards, on our own and by ourselves, sometimes in spite of ourselves and the system. We practise, and usually teach what we practice. The deeper we go, the deeper the experience and the results.

Science has monitored and wired practitioners, analysed their blood samples and studied behaviour to good effect. But science cannot measure the yoga experience. It cannot follow beyond subatomic particles into the actual *feeling*. This can only be felt, understood and described by the practitioner.

Erich Fromme writes: 'My faith in myself, in another, in humankind, in our capacity to become fully human also implies certainty, but certainty based on my own experience and not on my submission to an authority that dictates a certain belief' (Fromme 1976).

An Experiential Experiment

Past experience is useful for comparative practice, but there is no substitute for being in your experience as it *is* during practice. Past experience enables us to 'set things up' for immersion in the practice, but 'right now' experience is the guiding light as we observe tension, flux, texture and so on. Our experience is the practice as we meet sensations, feelings, ideas and insights. Immediate experience cannot be held, captured or taught. You cannot do anything with immediate experience other than let it guide you. Our own direct and immediate experience has always been and will always be the fundamental key to progress. Can we believe our own experience? To do so is the foundation for self-belief and authenticity. Students may be unsure of their own experience if the suggestions made are elusive. If feeling is 'sleepy', or well hidden, there may be confusion concerning what or how to feel. If conditioning is well established, it can take time for sensation to surface. For a while it may be necessary to take someone else's word that 'the feeling will come'.

For each of us our experience is our reality. Experience is defined in the Oxford English Dictionary as the fact of being consciously the subject of a state or condition. The 'yoga experience' is *on* when it is currently felt, and is in time with time. Experience flows as a movement. Experience is now; even when we refer to past experience, the reference is current.

The words *experience*, *experiment*, and *expert* come from the same Latin word *experientia*, meaning 'knowledge gained from repeated trials', and also stems from the word *periri*, meaning 'to go through'. Our expertise comes from going into and through our experience.

T.K.V. Desikachar, writing about his father in *The Yoga of Krishnamacharya* says:

'One of the striking things about his teaching is, whenever I ask him "Father, how did you get this information; where did you discover that, is it your own experience?" he will say, "No, it is my acarya; it is from my teacher." If someone asks where I [Desikachar] learnt something, my inclination is to say, 'This is my practise.' Now I know many things he [Krishnamacharya] tells are based on his own experience, but he will never acknowledge that. In fact, I asked him one day, "How is it you are able to say so much spontaneously?" He said, "I don't say those things; I close my eyes and it is the guru in me who says those things"' (Desikachar 1982).

Krishnamacharya's past experience served him well but this account from his son Desikachar implies that his spontaneity was founded on the movement of his current experience. The impersonality of his insights came through his direct experience of them.

If our perception of reality depends upon the quality and reliability of our own experience, it is preferable that the reality should be ours as opposed to someone else's. Our own reality is the authentic starting and finishing point; anything in between is, as Ramdass put it, 'Grist for the Mill' (Baba Ram Dass 1977).

R.D. Laing writes, 'It is not easy to say, even, what experience is. All experiences are instances of experiences but experience itself is not an experience' (Laing 1983). Laing suggests that there must be a stimulus to create an experience. We might interpret this as meaning that if there is no sensation to experience, there is no experience.

The fact that we are our experience provides us with the essential tool for deepening practice, i.e. our own irrefutable, immediate experience of what is happening takes us inward. Personal history may affect the clarity and sensitivity of experience, but if we get on with 'experiencing', it will enhance itself. The most advanced or most recent practitioners can only find it in themselves *at the time*. In this respect, there is no distinction between us.

We can, however, through certain practices, move beyond the experience of the practice and experience the phenomenon of experience. Some spiritual guides (Krishnamurti and others) refer to the possibility of having no experience at all, the ultimate emptiness. In this light, experience is seen as an addiction. But we need to experience something in order to anchor ourselves; it gives us security, even an unpleasant experience may be preferable to no experience at all. Chasing experiences is nothing new to yoga or life. We may spend considerable energy in trying to get back to where we were. The original experience of primal movement invites an experience from a pre-experiential time before conscious registration. Spontaneous movement is not guided by previous personal experience or modified by conditioning. But we do have the faculty of registration and recognition to evaluate and celebrate the experience. It is something we like to repeat; we are only human.

Experience is Feeling

Experience deepens as primal sensation awakens and we are given access to our origin. The experiment deepens as the body lets us in. All experience is felt. Everything that we are conscious of is felt, because consciousness itself is experience. Feeling is the bedrock of experience and the primary tool in practice.

Feeling is defined in the Oxford English Dictionary as 'a fact or state of consciousness' and in reality it is the fundamental tool of life because feeling is perception. Consciousness, feeling and experience are part of the same movement in time and combine to provide our sense of being that is often referred to as *isness*. 'Feeling' is physical, psychological and emotional, and usually combines all three simultaneously although we may not be aware of this. We can *have* a feeling, we can possess it

and we can *have* feeling generally, but at the same time we *are* feeling. Our entire experience of us is felt.

We perceive sensations or they remain beneath awareness to be processed by the organism. Activity that might be felt is frequently buried beneath awareness by conditioned patterns of tension. Feeling fully is a vital experience. We can experience ourselves vitally if we are going to shed more light on how we are. Vital is defined in the Oxford English Dictionary as 'essential to the existence of something absolutely indispensable'. Vitality through feeling is the principle of life; it is life.

Primitive man, in his innocence, may have felt a deep sense of *one with everything* but may not have *known* that he felt it. He was not tied to a *reflective* acuity that could disturb or enhance his original sensations. Sensory experience may well have provided the basis for the development of the brain and the mind that followed. Consciousness blossomed alongside the realisation of feeling. Feeling is the ancestor of thought.

Thought is our essential tool, but has taken over. Thought initially opens the door to the practice of yoga but is an impediment when it inhibits sensation. All sensation has its origin in primitive activity but not all primitive activity is sensed. A large proportion of physiological activity is not intended for awareness. Should it be, we would be overwhelmed by sensation, and unable to function.

The physiological properties of the spine and thoracic diaphragm contain sensory elements that are available to awareness and, when awoken, demonstrate the profound intelligence and power of the organism. Primal activity, and its sensation, reduces us to a state of 'less thought, more action' as involuntary movement is set free. The primal movement of the original body is the practice, the practitioner and the teacher.

Going Inward

When devotees gather before the Guru, it's not to feel him or her go inwards; they are there to feel him radiate outwards, emanate energy and being-ness. His powerful coming out-ness results from many years of going inward, from a deep inner exploration. As he radiates, a part of him continues to go inward; he unfolds. Our own experiment takes us inward. Introspection is fundamental to yoga practice. Self-observation and reflection form the bedrock for all practices. It is a quality requiring sensitivity.

Primal movement is an unfolding. We go in to come out; this is the art of practice. Going into the spine, sensing the vertebrae and the space between them, directing awareness to the deep pelvis, following the breath into an unknown inner space involves an inward movement of the mind. The mind enters and the body reveals its original nature. When we go in, we come out spontaneously and in tune with our *inness*. The spine and the breath reveal their primality.

It can take time to awaken deeper sensations; they may not arise easily and freely at first. The process is ongoing, but as we take part in it, the rewards are unexpected and profound. We can begin to experience an original state. An evolutionary blueprint carries the genetic experience of previous generations. Cellular memory provides a current account of behaviour that has taken millennia to evolve.

Following birth, intrauterine and birth experience excepted, we have no previous personal experience to speak of. It seems that the deeper we go, the further back in time we go. Spinal waves, preconscious states, womb-like or ancient experiences or fluid pulsations may be expressions of this.

Our true nature is founded upon the involuntary aspects of existence. True nature awakens when we acknowledge that it has no agenda and is responsive to our attention. Realisation is involuntary, but benefits from sensitive recognition. 'Without the inner the outer has no meaning, but without the outer the inner has no substance' (R.D. Laing, from a conversation with Jutta Laing).

Reduction

Reduction

*What comes to mind in someone whose spine begins
to move spontaneously for the first time: 'I'm reptilian,
snake like, a primal creature revealing itself through
the fog of my conditioning'. Sensations may range from
melting, 'I had no bones', 'I felt like a jelly fish', to 'I
felt like a collection of bones floating in a warm bath.'
These experiences highlight our organic and mechanical
heritage, demonstrate the co-dependence of these
properties, and are an unmistakable indication that we
are passing through habitual patterns. Practice takes us
into 'reduction'. We come back to an original state that
surfaces into awareness and takes over.*

The word *reduction*, from the Latin *reductionem*, means 'leading back or restoration (of a thing) to its origin, to restore to the truth, to bring back to a former state'. In medical terms, a sprain or fracture may be reduced; we also reduce habitual patterns or conditioning. We can reduce ourselves to a former condition, a clearer and freer way of being. Yoga explores reducibility, it looks at the possibility of reducing us to a preconditioned state. Practice potentially reduces the organism's negative patterns. Practice is reduction, and realising depth involves our capacity for reducibility.

Organisms and Mechanisms

We are, at one and the same time, and may feel like, organisms and mechanisms. Authorities on the human condition often use the word organism, a term used by scientists and spiritual teachers alike, to imply that beneath it all, beyond the veneer of personal conditioning and habit, lies an intelligence and a sensitivity common to all. Krishnamurti, Wilhelm Reich, Alexander Lowen and Albert Einstein, used the term 'organism'.

By organism we mean a living, animate, organic system. Do you feel like an organism during practice? The entire body is an organ made up of organs. The brain, spinal cord, diaphragm, soft tissue and skin come under the heading of organs. We can experience the spine as an organ as its wave-like movements lead us into a spontaneous inner dance that is beyond practice.

'Organism' implies sensitivity, intelligence, and it has a soft, fluid connotation. Reich suggested the organism has an innate need to express itself; we encounter expression as we go inward (Reich 1933). As we move through deeper levels we meet the expression of the organism, coming out from within. Inquiry and organic expression cross each other as a part of the unfolding movement of living tissue revealing itself.

The word 'mechanical' can have a more negative connotation. We may act, dance, make love and relate mechanically. Mechanical behaviour implies behaving without feeling. The organism's skeletal framework renders it mechanical in nature, but mechanical activity is sensed/felt organically. The organism is the 'feeler' through which we experience our mechanical aspects. We were organisms before we were mechanisms. In both evolutionary and embryonic terms, we have graduated from a cellular base bathed in fluid, to an organism that is mechanically supported and moved by a bony framework. The organisation of the framework has a direct bearing on the qualitative function of the organism.

A fundamental difference between the terms 'organism' and 'mechanism' is that the former describes something that *is* while the latter describes something that *happens* (although an organism is obviously happening). Organism tends towards involuntary activity and mechanism towards voluntary activity. We are organic but behave mechanically. But organic behaviour underpins mechanical behaviour. Our very substance is organic. Muscles act mechanically because of their organic properties – their substance.

Mechanics is intentionally divisive. Biomechanical approaches to the spine, pelvic and shoulder girdles et cetera highlight their working relationship under gravitational laws. Organics represents the organism as a whole, it is unifying.

Organic and mechanical properties are inseparable. Without the mechanical activity of the skeletal framework we may have remained an amorphous mass. We are how we are because we stood up and moved on land. The skeleton hardened out of soft organic tissue and fashioned itself in response to gravitational force and the upward thrust from the ground. Mechanics are provided by a system of uprights, levers, keystones, and arches, connected by articulations, moved by pulleys and guided by nervous activity.

Without the mechanical we would be a different life form, but without the organic we would be no life form at all. We are organic machines and mechanical organisms.

Mechanics are an inherent product of evolution and are ready for modification. Reducing our mechanical properties back to their original state (preconditioned) is assisted by nature. We did not *think up spinal curves*, nor did we *decide* that the best place for the roots of the diaphragm might be around the body's centre of gravity; we did not *think* our way into our relationship with the pull of the earth. Mechanical elements of balance have been *refining themselves* since we began to move on land. The art of practice is to uncover and encourage our inheritance.

Mechanical feelings involve joint movements. Performing postures and *positioning* is a mechanical activity. Feelings of organic softness, fluidity and pulsation arise as a consequence of mechanical application. For example, releasing tension by *reorganising* the long bones of the arms and legs in their relationship to the diaphragm and spine results in deep all–encompassing sensations of softness and fluidity. In practice, it is our organic nature that relays sensory information regarding tension and texture to awareness and enables us to adjust mechanically.

We 'do' the mechanical aspects of practice and benefit from the subsequent involuntary organic release and sensations. As a consequence of bony support, the yogi sitting in meditation can receive organic energy arising from deep within his pelvis and spine. We may sense our bones 'floating in fluid' (usually during rest periods but also at some stages of practising movement and postures) but the experience is provided by the organism.

In practice, we move back in time, beyond the mind and skeletal framework and into a pulsatile, warm, bath-like experience of an organism revealing itself.

Change is more profound when it follows natural mechanical and organic principles. Mechanical aspects need direction, while organic aspects need to be listened to. Allow your bones to breath inside the organic texture of your tissues.

The fact that we are organisms should be the first acknowledgement. We are organs and should treat ourselves accordingly. We would not throw the liver around, or ask it to perform things it has a resistance to, nor should we impose on the diaphragm, spine or the sacroiliac joints. When we slow down we can consider the need of the organism to be listened to. We have evolved from, and still are, organic creatures. We have been created; our most profound creativity may be found in the realisation of our creature-like nature. Allow your creature to come towards you.

Embryonic Sensations

'Paring back' can bring out sensations comparable to those that may be called embryonic. If one is interested in making this comparison there is certainly plenty of food for thought. *Re–experiences* may be re–lived during feelings of unfolding in practice. Embryonic growth may provide a template for adult experiences. The body-mind may release an embryonic memory. Such memories have been suggested by rebirthing practitioners, psychoanalysts and dream workers for many years. Reducibility may reveal sensational memories that we can associate with early growth formation.

When we give up control and surrender to forces that play through and emerge from within us, we can feel like and move like unfolding organisms, creatures or babies. An unchoreographed way of moving arises that feels perfectly natural. Some experiences may be described as intrauterine, and include feelings of unfolding, turning inside out, floating, complete fluidity, and the well-documented oneness with the environment. Such expression may resonate with primal experiences that predate cortical development and recapitulate the beginning of life as vertebrates. It is generally accepted by those involved in bodywork that these experiences arise as a consequence of releasing tension. The depth of the experience is synonymous with the depth of the release.

Some interesting studies have been conducted by Jaap van der Wal, a Dutch embryologist at Maastricht University in Holland. The results of his research into a connection between embryological growth and inherent spirituality are convincing and also relevant to the deeper yoga experience. He explores prenatal development in order to show how biology expresses the essence of spiritual development and unfolding. The following observations are published in his paper 'Speech of the Embryo' (2003). For our purposes I have reiterated and highlighted some of his observations and their implications.

He writes:

Bodily functions, physiological functions, psychological functions, are pre-exercised as growth gestures and growing movements in the embryo. In this respect a human being has already breathed long before he has taken his first breath after birth. The dynamics in the sense of the gesture of morphological development – with which lungs, thorax, and diaphragm unfolding, may be considered and interpreted as a type of breathing because they are breathing movements. The breathing of an embryo is not yet breathing air in a physiologic way, but it represents a more fundamental breathing in a morphological way, in form so to speak. Considered this way, an embryo looks, grasps, walks. It also stands on its feet and holds its own. The gesture and action of stretching and standing upright is already being performed or pre-exercised by the human embryo in the fifth to the tenth week of prenatal development as a gesture of growth. This standing during growth is a necessary condition for a developing body, a being that later on is able to stand and go upright physiologically and even psychologically.

The following aspects of intrauterine growth, highlighted by Jaap van der Wal, resonate with the primal movement experience:

- Embryological development is a 'gesture' (a gesture is an expression and gestation implies emergence, formation, coming into being).

- The centre of the 9-day-old embryo doesn't move; movement and growth occur around the centre.

- In the first few weeks, the embryo is reaching outwards from a centre around which all activity revolves, like a wheel around an axis.

- There are two tendencies in early embryonic development: a connecting tendency and a space-making tendency.

- In the first week, the embryo shows tendencies of consolidation, with motion towards its centre. In the second week, the opposite occurs, an opening towards the periphery (centring precedes expansion).

- Within the third week, there is a gathering up of the inner body.

- Body cavities are organs; they are activities and active.

- It appears that the human embryo, because of its process of differentiation, falls into various constituents and parts, and that the embryo at the same time centres this process.

- Our extremities come out of the ventral (front) aspect of the embryo.

- The dorsal (back) side is where we implant into the womb.

- Animal life's first gesture is to grow in; plants grow out.

- The front (ventral) and back (dorsal) move towards each other; the front moves back and the back moves forward, they come together.

- At first, the umbilical cord is dorsal (at the back).

- The embryo grows out of itself.

- In the first embryonic week, only the dimension of space is present.

- In the first week, what will become the head and pelvis begin to separate and the spine begins to appear between them. A rhythmic process between head and pelvis reveals the spine.

- In the fourth week, the head and pelvis emerge from the rounded preliminary embryo — unfolding. The head grows towards its eventual position and the neck is formed. It is an unfolding, as the rolled-up embryo opens out. The process is repeated in post-natal development. The head goes up first, then the baby sits up, the pelvis turns under the trunk and this leads to standing. It is as if the embryonic unfolding was a rehearsal for unfolding within the gravitational field.

- In the fourth week, the dorsal expands and the front moves in, i.e. the back comes round to the front so that the dorsal becomes the whole outside of the body.

- In the fourth week come the first autonomous gesture and individuation. This demonstrates that the gesture of growth, how we move, the quality of expression predating any kind of mechanical law, is more fundamental than the mechanics of movement.

- The full-term baby births itself.

We may posit from the work of Jaap van der Wal and in relation to sensations encountered in depth practice that:

- The human figure has come forth from movement.

- The forces that formed the body are at work throughout life and carry the blueprint of health into manifestation at every moment — embryonic behaviour can be interpreted as human behaviour.

- We can feel like *adult embryos* — the body's form and shape can be felt and seen as a basic behaviour, an expression of primality.

Unfolding

Evolution is an unfolding of life. From everything that is 'known' about embryological and evolutionary development, we can say that we have unfolded. The word *evolve* means to unfold, it comes from the Latin *evolvere*, meaning 'to bring out what exists implicitly

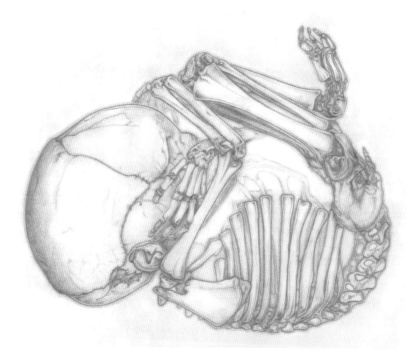

Figure 2.1

This basic image of a fetal framework gives a strong sense of our enfoldment in utero. A truly primal attitude.

or potentially'. This interpretation provides an intelligent basis for practice and teaching. Evolution implies 'the process of developing from a rudimentary to a complete state'. Evolution is the fundamental process of the movement of unfolding. Unfolding is an evolutionary gesture of growth and we tap into its blueprint in practice. Unfolding is also defined as an 'unwinding in a spiral form', an experience common in practice. Figure 2.1 portrays the enfoldment of the human framework in utero.

Unfolding relates to all biological/physiological activity. The cells, embryo, limbs, and spine unfold. Consciousness is an unfolding of awareness. Our deepest nature is represented by an uninhibited outward movement of unfolding. The fixed form is always the end result of the process of movement, i.e. we unfold into the material representation of ourselves. 'The organism gestures itself into existence – the physical specifications for the mature organism crystallised out of gesturing' (Jaap van der Wal).

Continued success of an organism in any habitat implies that its structural/functional organisation is complementary to features of its environment, and they can only be studied intelligently together, that is, as one system. Indeed, some hold that the various control systems of an organism necessarily embody a 'model' of their environment for effective responses to occur (Gray's Anatomy 1989).

Gravitation and breathing give perfect examples of the above statement; they also combine as the two primary factors in practice. Whatever the biological/physiological details of evolution, these basic elements are essential for deepening the yoga experience. Even more relevant is the fact that they are primary responses to our environment. The areas needing the most work, the spine, diaphragm and their associates, tend to be poor responders to their habitat as a consequence of habit. A substantial portion of habit is usually centred on spinal fixations and the breath.

We have left the ocean and the womb and unfolded from the ground. We experienced gravity at the same time that our blood received oxygen from the surrounding air. We were vertebrates in water and then on land. The diaphragm developed as a primary breathing muscle on land but is also a postural muscle. The spine is not only an organ of support but also an organ of respiration. The attachment between the spine and the diaphragm is particularly relevant. The spine provides an essential anchor for the diaphragm and the diaphragm in turn supports and also frees the spine. We can feel them in practice as one organ or mechanism.

When we pare it back, our original behaviour in practice has an involuntary component and mirrors early essential responses to gravity, respiration and the impulse to move, aided by our purchase on the ground (the uterine walls).

Further to this is an impulse to expand outwards from within, a familiar sensation in practice. Deeper experiences may be memories of *growth experiences* or *gestures* relating to an embryonic or evolutionary blueprint. Sensations may include fluidity, melting, waves, floating, drawing inwards and expansion. The more sensitive we become, the deeper we find ourselves within our own organism. Our interest may be weighted towards the development of the species or towards more personal embryonic possibilities. The personal is only a generation away. Intrauterine growth happened in our lifetime and, all things equal, we know our host. On the other hand, on an evolutionary basis we are continuing to unfold in time with time. (See time as movement!!) This has connotations for 'being in the present'; the movement of life is never in the present. Life moves from past to future through the present.

Unfolding from the Ground

The Primary Force

> *How would it have felt, that first contact with land, washed ashore, an ancient creature registering pressure, weight and inertia as gravity bore down, holding it back, inhibiting its fluidity. We unfolded into our environment with the earth as our purchase.*

Practice cannot escape gravity; it represents our mechanical roots. The organism had to invest in mechanics to move and stand up on land. Primal movement, the deep body, and how and what we feel, are the consequence of the earth's pull. We are constantly reminded of gravity as we work. 'The weight going down' is recognised by many practitioners. The points are: firstly, not to underestimate gravity's power from the beginning; secondly, to what extent can and does weight go down; and thirdly, how to use it. We are programmed not to feel our own weight due to our upward response, but when lifting someone we are clearly reminded of an inertia that we have successfully overcome.

As far as gravity is concerned, there are only two movements: towards and way from the ground. The spine is encouraged to lengthen. The upward movement involves lightness, freedom and a deep inner strength that arises from within the articulations as they open. Contact with the ground is reinforced by the deep unfolding of the frontal spine from the middle of the lumbar and lower thoracic vertebrae. The gravity experience is considerable, sobering and enlightening.

Fashioned by Gravity

Anatomy and physiology has been fashioned by gravity. Every bone, tissue and cell is the way it is because of the body's attempt to counter gravitation. We naturally resist gravity and respond to its force through the mechanical support of an articulated skeleton and reflexive soft tissue.

Poor gravitation takes its toll: Irvin Korr, a leading pioneer in osteopathic research, observed: 'Although the importance of the relationship between gravity and bodily structure is thoroughly recognised in osteopathic practice, our knowledge of the interplay of those relationships is too fragmentary to provide a basis for the *prevention* (my italics) of the initiation of the process so important to the prevention of functional and organic disease' (Korr 1951). Korr acknowledges the importance of the quality of gravitation but admits to uncertainty regarding the mechanical activity involved.

Around the same time, pioneers of the gravity–health relationship, notably Mabel Todd, Moshe Feldenkrais and Ida Rolf, had been making discoveries of their own to good effect. Classic osteopathy (as opposed to the more medically disposed branch of the profession) had been proposing a particularly sophisticated approach to biomechanical principles in the gravitational field. This approach involved a complex study of keystones, pivots, spinal arches, curves and several gravity lines that might draw our attention away from the organic nature of spinal activity.

In our practice, we are not attempting to fit into an ideal *model* of gravitation. Personal patterns vary and the nature of our work promotes a spontaneously intelligent response as we progress. Beneath the personal patterns, we tend to respond in a similar way but may express it differently as we unfold from the ground. Someone may have so-called perfect alignment but be stiff and ill at ease in their body and exhibit a poor response in a variety of positions. Another person may be relatively crooked yet gravitate deeply, moving with extreme lightness and grace. Vanda Scaravelli was a good example of this. She had a marked spinal scoliosis, but the freedom between her bones, her contact with the earth and extraordinary lightness and deep strength gave the impression of a creature with deep roots yet unfettered by weight. We can feel inseparable from the earth's pull and cultivate our response. We are organic aspects of a gravitational field.

Some Lines and Centres

The fundamental principles regarding human gravitation confirm what our body tells us. We have been moulded by gravity and you can see from the body's bony framework that its response has been extraordinary. Skeletal shape, the nature of the articulations, the intelligent design of the spine and its curves, its relationship to the thorax and to the long bones through the upper and lower girdles are a tribute to natural engineering.

The three primary forces to be aware of are:

1 the downward pull of the earth,
2 the upward thrust from the ground, and
3 the living responsive force of the body.

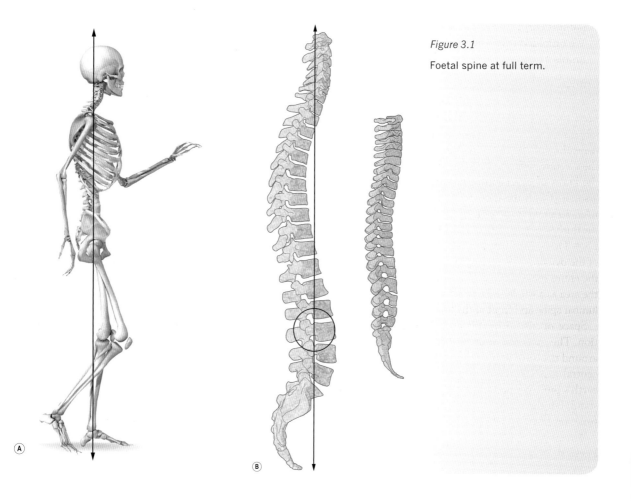

Figure 3.1

Foetal spine at full term.

(A)

(B)

At its simplest, biomechanical ideas on gravitation propose the following: Figure 3.1 shows the basic gravity line and center of gravity. A foetal spine indicates the beginning of natural spinal curves.

- A hypothetical gravity line (GL) runs through the centre of gravity (COG). The gravity line is the result of all forces that play through body. It falls from the odontoid process of the axis through the sacral promontory, medial to the hip and knee to the talonavicular joint.

- The COG is an imaginary point around which all parts of the body balance each other. The GL, or line of weight, passes through the centre of gravity. The location of the centre of gravity changes considerably and may locate outside the body depending on the arrangement of its parts. Practicing postures and movements makes it impossible to predict where the COG or the GL are at any given time, but it is useful to know where it locates in standing. We unfolded from the earth and needed a centre to unfold from.

When we stand, the middle of the lumbar curve is the osteopathic COG. Standard biomechanical theory positions the COG lower down at the front of the second sacral segment. Both centres are relevant and both shift depending on the position of the body. You can visualise these centres when standing and loosely gravitating with the knees slightly flexed. The osteopathic centre is more associated with the thoracic diaphragm, and its dynamic relationship to the middle of the waist. This area includes the third lumbar vertebrae and the discs between L2/3 and L3/4. The centre in front of the sacrum is relevant because of the dynamic relationship between the sacral curve and the entire spine above it. The important thing is to sense the area as a whole – the front of the sacrum through the lumbar spine and front of the lower thoracic area.

Space opens up in this area during healthy gravitation. The potential of the human framework is centred around the third lumbar disc. It is the part of the body's central axis that has adapted most successfully to the earth's pull. We needed the purchase of the ground to stand, but the central lumbar area enabled the spine to function in an upright position.

When you unfold from a forward bend with the knees slightly flexed, you can feel the strength in this area and its dynamic spread in two directions towards the ground and head.

As we unfolded, the biggest change came at the pelvis as the front of the hip joints opened and the pelvis moved from a horizontal to a more vertical alignment, but the spine had to accommodate and take part in unfolding, hence the development of the spinal curves which are suited for balancing and distributing the weight of the body.

The 11th and 12th thoracic vertebrae are said to represent the front and upper support of the body and provide the main point of resistance to the weakening of the spinal curves. You can *feel* this area open in conjunction with the front of the lumbar spine in practice and its action feeds the entire body down into the arches of the feet and up into the jaw. The above confirms that the dynamic support and opening that we can feel through the front of the mid-lumbar and lower thoracic spine is relevant to practice and that these areas should be courted in awareness.

The Reliable Perpendicular

The information we are given by authorities on biomechanics is useful, relevant and affirming. We know, by feeling it in ourselves, that balance and stability are maximised when the base of support is large, when the centre of gravity is close to the base, and when weight passes through the body as close to the gravity line as possible. We know this because, in many positions involving standing or sitting, we have learnt to drop our weight, open the base, contain our limbs and organise our head to minimise tension.

Practice has its own agenda. We can abandon our weight and respond naturally without analysis. We don't need to think about centres of gravity or central gravity lines. When the body is in the throes of deep action, its responses to gravity are revealed in a way that is beyond analysis and external frames of reference. As we unwind and express a deeper action, the body will move as it pleases. Any return to 'lines and centres' will be spontaneous. Gravity passes through the body at a 90° angle to the ground that is constant regardless of position. Body weight continually shifts and adjusts itself around a perpendicular line, not only through large movements, but also through breathing movements and general subtle oscillations and waves. Our frame of reference concerns what and how we perceive tension and the quality of action. All contact points with the ground in any position, directly feed the spine as it returns to its primal nature.

Contact Points

We directly feel our contact points with the earth. The body organises itself gravitationally in relation to where we touch the ground. How we organise and sense our contact points with the ground provides a major influence on gravitation. Depending on position, any bony area acts a gravitation point. Imagining one or more plumb lines running at a 90° angle through any of the contact points you may choose in any position gives an additional dimension to the use and distribution of weight. Gravity lines always pass through the body's contact points with the ground and are always perpendicular to it, i.e. at a 90° angle in any and all positions.

Whatever the point of contact, knee, hip, pelvis, spine, elbow, heel, et cetera, the gravity line passes through at the same angle; it is only the position of the body that changes.

Contact points provide a conduit for the two-way movement, towards and away from the ground; for example, when unfolding from all fours, your ankles and wrists can open and receive weight going through them from above, and the thrust from the ground moving in the opposite direction. This is where the space, lightness and inner strength come from.

These imaginary lines are a simple factor in practice because the contact points that they pass through are so easily and immediately felt. A responsive spine 'picks up' the upward thrust from the ground. We can position the bones in a way that maximises gravitation.

For example, when we lay on our backs the spine actively receives weight passing through the spinal vertebrae in contact with the ground, i.e. the mid-thoracic area and the sacrum. The middle of the lumbar and cervical curves may respond by lifting. Maximising the feel of a contact point may have an effect locally and also remotely, e.g. consolidating the contact point between the right pelvis and ground will open the left shoulder through the agency of the spine.

Resisting the Earth

The word 'gravitation' should not only imply weight going down but should include in its meaning our upward movement as an immediate response. Going towards and away from the earth are part of the same thing.

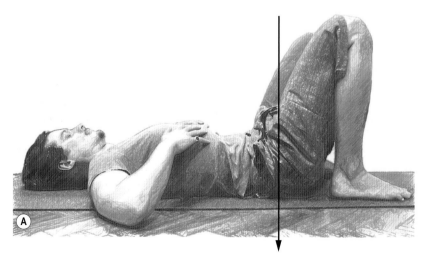

Figure 3.2A

Contact point and gravity line — through the pelvis.

A

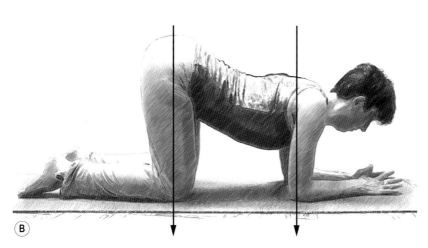

Figure 3.2B

Contact points and gravity lines — through the elbow and knee.

Bones provide the essential contact (given that they are sleeved in tissue) with the ground. But the gravitational experience brings to life the responsive force of the organism, which is filtered through complex and integrated sets of sensory motor reactions within the soft tissues. Tissues sense the tension, and their most basic reactions are simple involuntary reflexes taking place beneath a conscious level. The most frequently cited is the stretch reflex, which guides and controls soft tissue activity in relation to gravitation. The weight of the body literally stretches the sensory nerves in the muscles, which stimulate the motor nerve of the muscles to contract and support our weight. It is well known that the stretch reflex can be weakened by pulling and overstretching muscles and it is generally realised that listening to the body's sensations enhances sensitivity and tissue efficiency. The tissue tensing sense might be the most ancient property inherent in animal life. Tissue tension gives a sense of self. We are a response to our environment, essentially gravity, which provides the organism with a tensional reflexive nature. Tension is a primary sensation but in the early stages of evolution there would have been no neo-cortex for the conscious registration of this sense. All movement necessitates tension and its release, The organism would have registered this somewhere inside itself.

The tensegrity view suggests that the body is held together by elements that are also trying to pull it apart and that the resultant tension holds us up against the force of gravity. This concept suggests that bone and soft tissue (myofascia) work together to provide an inner tension that simultaneously centres and expands us in order to resist gravity. In the embryo, the growing bones (preformed in cartilage) push outwards from the core acting as rods that reinforce the action of soft tissues. The tissues are lengthened under tension by the ongoing expansion of the bones, and also hold the bones back against the central axis of the body, creating an inner supportive tension. This working arrangement continues from infancy into adulthood and can be utilised in practice.

Tensegrity can be *felt* when we become sensitive enough and is one of the enlightening sensations produced by deepening practice. The long bones of the limbs are attracted towards and away from the central axis of the spine through the pelvic and shoulder girdles.

The body is also gravity resistant through its fluid content. The physiological picture changes when we consider and experience the potential of our deep fluid nature. This aspect of practice will be covered in more depth in Chapter 13. We are at least 80 per cent fluid, which is gravity resistant. We can view (and feel) ourselves as fluid containers bound by skin. A suitable analogy might be the rubber hot-water bottle, flaccid and compressible when empty but firm and pressure resistant when full.

The major cavities of the body are also resistant to external pressure as a result of their internal pressure.

The abdominal cavity is packed with organs, and is bounded by the pelvic floor, thoracic diaphragm, abdominal and belly muscles, all contributing to an inner resistance. The thoracic cavity contains an element of residual air, and the negative pressure between the pleura of the lungs and the inner thoracic walls provide the chest with an inner resistance to external forces.

In effect, we resist gravity in a variety of ways, some perhaps more applicable than others depending, on the moment and the focus during the immediacy of practice. We can appreciate the whole body as a gravity-resistant organ, an animate spring that counters its own weight by actively responding to the forces that draw it downwards.

Gravity in the East

West or East, the gravity and the ground are the same but the response differs. The Eastern appreciation of gravity is non-scientific. Easterners are 'in gravity' and consequently have not studied it in our mechanical terms.

The Eastern body has maintained its primal roots well. Looking down at a group of Eastern feet, you notice that apart from size there is little difference between them. The feet are generally broad anteriorly, and have large heels and open space between the toes. They contact the earth where they should, at the outer back heel and at the base of the greater and little toes, presenting efficient, pliable, triangular bases for receiving the upward thrust from the ground. The benefits of an intelligent base reflect upward. Ankles and knees show space, the spinal curves are shallow and confluent, and the upper body appears relatively light and free. Individual discrepancies notwithstanding, the Eastern relationship to gravity is impressive.

The yoga masters knew about the energetic connection between thought and physical tension and understood that it took considerable energy to sustain rampant mental activity. They understood how energy, trapped at the upper end of the system, needed to be earthed. They knew that energy takes the line of least resistance and

that dropping their weight drained tension and informed their personal inquiry. They gave their weight away, sensitively inviting an ascendance of energy to move upward.

The word Guru also means one who is very heavy, heavy with energy, heavy like a pregnant woman, heavy with the unknown, heavy with the divine.

Osho (Osho 1996)

Using the Ground

The fact that the earliest humans lived close to the earth would have been reflected in the quality of their gravitation. They were at the later stages of unfolding and their contact with the earth would have been well consolidated and unimpaired by a complex and busy neocortex. Thinking and its excesses would not have pulled up their roots. A reconsideration of gravitation in practice is essential for deepening a sense of unfolding and exposing our potential for a natural and powerful expression. Using the ground has inestimable value for reducing habitual patterns, for reaching inwards towards the depth body, and for returning to a state that existed pre-yoga, before yoga had been thought of. Deepening contact with the earth takes time; it is a gradual process. One of our biggest fears may well be one of abandonment, but the ground will never withdraw its support.

This preliminary practice is a gravitational reminder. It uses lying down to reduce the influence of postural reflexes (see figures 3.3A-B). The effects are mainly spinal but the entire system takes part. Although the body has a self-organising inherency, it may need some initial direction.

From time to time, as sensation dictates, reorganise your bones in relation to the ground and to each other to release tension and maximise the effects. There is no 'when' to this; let sensitivity guide you. At times, the gravitational responses weaken and you may need to reconsider your contact points. Shifting your weight just several inches sometimes can reinvigorate the process. You cannot teach this aspect but you can encourage its exploration:

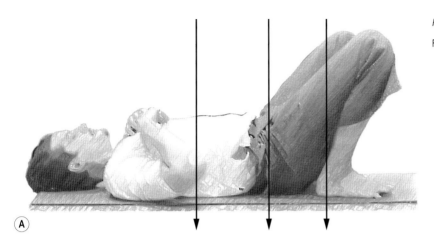

Figure 3.3A

Face up.

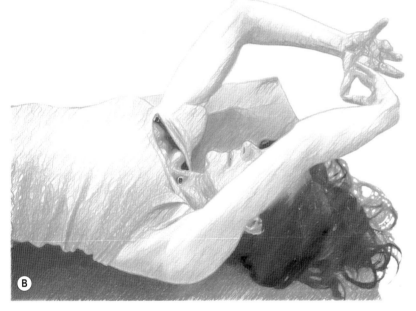

Figure 3.3B

Expressing the arms.

- To begin with, use your basic understanding of the skeletal framework to visualise and sense the shape of your bones and articulations. Feel and think *into* your body. You will notice how you let go of *thought feelings* and *feeling thoughts* begin take over. You may find yourself yielding entirely to the ground and to your sensations while superfluous thought idles in the background or dissolves entirely.

- Be gently attentive, opening yourself to possibilities.

- Be heavy through your contact points.

- This process is not passive, and although at first we should relax, a deeper activity becomes more apparent and more dynamic. We have not evolved through relaxation. The physiology of evolution and intrauterine life is dynamic. Relaxation is certainly a component and we keep coming back to it, but we do so in order to release muscular conditioning and habit. Allow your impulse to move to be stimulated by a deeper involuntary action.

- Giving your weight to the ground will activate your breath; as your exhalation spontaneously deepens you will gravitate more deeply.

- *Become a creature*; know less and feel more, give yourself up to something larger than you.

- How you organise yourself is based on what you feel. Disengage your external muscles and engage with your spine. *You can only find it in yourself.* This may involve alternating between positions, lifting your head, turning it, releasing your jaw, placing the ball of the foot and or toe on the wall, opening the centre of the feet, allowing the long bones of the arms to drop back into their sockets to release the spine through the girdles. Explore the possibilities of release and gravitation when on your side or half turned to the side.

- Become small and soft; contain yourself. Let gravity pass through you. The possible arrangements are numerous. Rearranging the configuration of the long bones activates the spine from various angles.

- *Try new contact points* — some within inches of each other — and explore the ground through your contact points and invite imaginary gravity lines through them.

- Gravity lines pass through your limbs and your spinal curves, and open the middle of the lumbar spine, and stimulate your thoracic spine.

- Cultivate a *sense* of the depth of your lumbar curve.

- Keep abandoning your contact points to the earth, surrender to them.

- Let the back of your waist go down as you exhale, feel it spread in all directions, feel it come up again as you inhale.

- Minimise muscular support and maximise skeletal support. When we sink to release and release to sink, when conditioning yields, we are 'sucked in' and strengthened from the ground and from within.

- Let go to the ground; drop, drop, and drop again until the action of dropping becomes a continual movement of falling, in time with time — follow the path of least resistance, rediscover a primal state.

- Your entire spine and your mind can respond to total gravitation; there is no method.

We can return to this practice time and again, as a process in itself or as a preparation for other work. The degree of tension held by the system and the quality and depth of its response to gravity are inseparable. Habitual tension is dissolved by gravitation. Practice is deepened by returning to the earth. Your spine, through millions of years of evolution, understands gravity more deeply than biomechanical authority, and more profoundly than you do. Gravity and contact with earth have fashioned the spine and it has responded by becoming part of the gravitational field. This is a beginning!

The way of love is not a subtle argument
The door there is destruction
Birds make great sky circles of their freedom
How do they do this?
They fall
And in falling they are given wings.

Rumi (Barks 1997)

Tension: The First Feeling

Your Tension

We are inspired by new sensations. The quality of sensation depends on how we work with tension. Tension is the first feeling because feeling is tension.

Gross and fine sensation arising into consciousness is a consequence of tensional activity. Thinking, feeling and consciousness are tension. Even bliss is tension because it exists. Existence is tension, we *are* tension; we are a condensation of energy bound by tension. Each one of us is a matrix of organic tissue held together by tension; we are a contraction.

Practice involves engaging, avoiding, releasing, using or modifying tension to enhance the quality of the work. Tension constantly changes texture depending on how we feel or think. The intelligence and sensitivity of tension renders it unpredictable, even when conditions are ideal. Tension is the first feeling in practice because tension *is* feeling. Sensation is provided by the tensional receptivity of sensory nerves.

Tension may have been our earliest feeling, giving us sensations of expansion, contraction, movement, and a general sensation of being alive. These feelings had no higher consciousness within which to register (as far as we can tell). In practice we immerse into primal sensations of tension but with an evolved awareness enabling us to recognise and evaluate their texture. Feelings of tension may take us back to a physiological beginning. When we negotiate with tension we engage with ancient intelligence.

The Movement of Tension

All movement is tension on the move. Breathing movements, wave-like movements, oscillations and pulsations reflect a rhythmicity of tension moving through the body, taking part in the dance of life. The entire body resembles a versatile tensional spring that accommodates and is responsive to gravity and movement.

As we activate deeper tensional qualities they move outwards to release the enveloping tension of habit and conditioning; the inner passes through the outer. The waves of tension and release, felt and seen on the surface of the body, come from deep primal activity expressing itself.

Tension in the body applies to all tissue, but our interest in tension is predominately myofascial. The Oxford English Dictionary defines tension as, 'the action of being stretched' from the stem of the Latin '*tendere*' stretch, hence the term *tense* grity with regard to stretching out from a central axis.

Tension is also defined as 'the condition, in any part of the body of being stretched or strained; a sensation indicating or suggesting this; a feeling of tightness' and 'a straining or strained condition, of the mind feelings, or nerves'. In physics tension implies a constrained condition of the particles of a body when subjected to forces acting in opposite directions away from each other (usually along the body's greatest length), thus tending to draw them apart, balanced by forces of cohesion holding them together. Cohesion is also tension in the opposite direction.

We have learnt to respect tension, not only as an indication of force or as a guide, but also to respect its information, what it is telling us, how it makes us feel, and the fact of its long-standing intelligence.

Personal and Primal Tension

Tension is best understood by experiencing its resistance, elasticity, and the immediacy of its aliveness. You are your tension and your tension is you. All tensional feelings are personal, as they register in the consciousness of the person feeling them. But there is a distinction between patterns installed by personal history and those that are species originated. The former may grip, divide, and restricts sections of the body, while the latter integrates, opens, moves and strengthens the body from within. Primal tension overlaid by personal tension gives you your sense of you.

Tissue tension sense sets the tone of 'feeling ourselves'. If you and I exchanged soft tissue we would feel like different people; the unaccustomed tissue contains a record of unfamiliar personal history. In some, the patterns would differ so much it would be impossible to function on any level. If Beethoven had suddenly acquired an alternative pattern, the results would have been disastrous. Hitler's patterns proved calamitous and a change might have been beneficial. Individual patterns are essential and are the spice of life, but enmeshed within them lie networks of tension connected to past experience that may or may not be advantageous.

Practice can feel as if we are trying to *get into or out of* ourselves, often at the same time. As the body unfolds, it is as if we are turning inside out or outside in. The entire organism expresses itself outwardly and inwardly through tension. The unfolding of the deeper body is a prolific expression of mechanical and organic tension. This may be comparable to the much more powerful tension of birth and orgasm. Practice is neither, but it can sometimes feel as if we pass through, into and out of a transformative physiological state. Babies exhibit substantial tension as they explore themselves and their environment. They look as if they are *trying to get out of themselves*. And indeed they are as they break out of a primal pattern

that holds them close to their centre, an essential prerequisite for growth and development.

Towards and Away From

In life, everything moves towards and away from a centre, a simultaneous tension of attraction and distraction. This polarity depends on balanced tension between poles. A cell moves towards and away from its nucleus, blood moves towards and away from the heart, cerebrospinal fluid moves towards and away from its productive centre in the brain, nervous conduction flows towards and away from the central nervous system. Embryological development involves an unfolding towards and away from a centre. Consciousness is a movement towards and away from our environment. Some structures invaginate; i.e. turn in on themselves.

Muscle activity involves a tension towards and away from the muscle belly. The tension of tensegrity involves a polarised tension towards and away from the spine. The body moves towards and away from the earth. We move (emotionally) towards and away from each other, sometimes within the same moment. The tension between us holds us together and apart.

At its simplest we are an ongoing rhythmic process of contraction and expansion, towards and away from a centre. The efficiency of this process is determined by elasticity, power and fluidity in both directions. Introversion is the first stage of opening up — we go in to come out, unfolding is one movement made up of intro- and extroverting — like opening a pair of socks. Thus introversion is the tensional action of drawing inwards and unfolding from your deep body. As we restore the natural interplay of poles, the organism finds an original balance.

Feeling Tension

Our executive organs, the muscles, the engines of movement, constantly moving between tension and release, are controlled by a delicate and sensitive arrangement of structures, neurons and chemicals. Muscle can only tense or release, and the relevant physiology is extensive and available in many good texts.

We cannot feel the cellular mechanics or chemistry of tension; we feel the tension itself. It is of little help to suggest texture to sarcomeres, myofibrils, actin, myosin or nerve end plates. Thinking about adrenaline and endorphin secretion (although we do) does not necessarily assist us with tension negotiation. The chemistry and finer mechanics of neuromuscular tension is interesting and can be useful but you cannot feel this activity, it takes place beneath a conscious level. If the reverse were true we would be flooded with information and be unable to feel clearly. Information that is unfeelable adds to knowledge, but in practice knowledge is a tension that has lost fluidity. It is more useful to acknowledge (*acknowledgement* meaning 'knowledge through recognition') the distinction between personal and primal tension and the potential for refining their relationship.

When you are *in it*, you are *in it*! You are in the changes of tone and texture, you are in the aliveness that tells you that tension moves, opens, releases, circulates, and returns like a creature with an unpredictable nature. You are in a sensory cocktail of gathering, opening, softening, spreading, grounding and lifting. You are a witness to, and subject of, an inner dance with expression as the only agenda.

Expressing and Repressing Tension

Tension is activity that is either denied or allowed expression. The body expresses or represses tension. Movement is an expression of tension and a lack of movement reflects its repression. In the 1930s and 1940s, at the time that B.K.S. Iyengar was beginning to develop his approach to yoga in Southern India, Wilhelm Reich, at first in Germany and then in the USA, was pioneering the inclusion of body work in psychoanalysis. Reich recognised that addressing chronic patterns of tension was essential in helping his patients to resolve their issues. Their two major works, *Light on Yoga* (Iyengar), and *Character Analysis*

(Reich) could not be further apart, culturally or in their methodology, but each in their own way, seriously and thoroughly, approached the problem of body-mind tension.

Reich's approach to repressive tension was radical. A contemporary of Freud and a psychoanalyst and sex counsellor, he took the concept of tension and emotion further than anyone had until that time. He was one of the first to propose that emotional expression is held back by chronic tension in the skeletal muscles and pointed out that repressed emotional activity developed a muscular armouring, indicating that the tension of fear is not only produced by external threats but also by a fear of feeling unwanted and potentially overwhelming emotions. Reich writes: 'The patient first had to establish contact with himself before he could grasp the connection between his various neurotic mechanisms. As long as the armour functioned, the patient could at best achieve only an intellectual comprehension of his situation. According to experience, this had minor therapeutic effect' (Reich 1933). The experience of body workers, movement teachers, postural re-educators and yoga teachers confirms the correspondence between tissue texture and unexpressed emotion. Iyengar's approach, also radical in its own way, focused on simply 'doing the work'. One worked hard with the body-mind allowing the emotional content to take care of itself. This is not to say Iyengar was not compassionate; he was.

Going inwards is as expressive as moving outwards and is expressed as a feeling in many forms of dance. The point is not to stay in, but to be aware of the need to expand as a reflection of the primal movement of unfolding. The outer body is not a passive recipient of inner expression but exhibits the movement coming from within.

Patterning

Individual patterns of unresolved tension superimpose on to primary tension. Tension holds us in our body and glues our emotional, psychological and physiological elements.

Reich writes: 'A person's character is the functional sum total of all past experience' (1942). He continues:

In the final analysis I could not rid myself of the impression that somatic rigidity represents the most essential part in the process of repression. All our patients report that they went through periods in childhood, in which by means of certain practices in vegetative behaviour (holding the breath, tensing the abdominal muscular pressure, etc.) they learned to suppress their impulses of hate, anxiety and love. ... it can be said that every muscular rigidity contains the history and meaning of its origin.

Individual patterns may grip anywhere or everywhere. Sometimes, the entire organism appears to be in a state of shock. Tension may affect the jaw, mouth, eyes, neck, throat, chest, spine, abdomen, shoulders or diaphragm. Deeper, more protected areas as well as surface areas may be bound up and their relationship disturbed. Joints may be habitually pulled together, including spinal segments and their curves. The legs may be pulled into the pelvis, the pelvis into the spine,

Patterns may be one-sided. Everyone has a weak, or more held side, and an imbalance between sides may stem from a variety of causes. Generally, everyone has a scoliosis. (See Ch. 15: 'The Original Spine'). One side of the body may be more expressive and the other side more repressed. We can work for a more harmonious balance between sides.

As we move into deeper tension and exchange our dependency on external muscular support for a stronger internal support, we pass through emotional patterns of tension. As the spine and its associates awaken, old patterns tend to be pushed outwards, and although they reoccur, are generally weaker, have less power, and are supported by a deeper sense of self. Surrendering the body to a deeper place gives insight into dissolving the self generally and this can be well supported by deeper feelings of physical strength and fluidity. In time, the transformation can be surprising.

Attachment to Tension

We may be attached or even addicted to our tensional patterns because they represent who we are. We are attached *to* our muscular settings because we are attached *by* them, they hold *us* together and we may even reinforce them in practice. We tend to foster a subtle addiction to our identity. Dissolving the tension that provides us with our sense of self may take time. Some patterns are obvious from the start while others take time to reveal themselves. Habitual activity may be too well established to step aside for long. A small shift away from the culture of the 'me' is considerable progress. Surrendering non-essential tension in small bursts may be good enough; effects are incremental, and time provides a more sustained transformation.

In the unlikely event of abandoning all personal tension at once, we might weep, laugh, rock, cling or dance, but the deep centre of the body and the ground provide effective anchors. Tension often releases following a deeper practice. Dreams, insight or surges of affection are commonplace and *surfacing* of any kind is generally supported by an inner strength. *As tensions release we are supported by a deeper, less-conditioned tension that takes over, enabling the outer patterns to let go.*

It is as if two creatures are present, an acquired creature that lives upon us, and an inherent creature that emerges from within us when conditions are favourable. Releasing the outer tension reveals a powerful and ancient tension. If you have ever held a snake, you will have experienced the power in your hands. The muscular action of a snake is strong; its spinal anatomy is not unlike ours. Snakes move with great agility and from a deep strength coming from the relay of muscles extending throughout the length of their exclusively spinal bodies.

Working with Tension

Tension feeds the experience of practice. We can let go relatively but never completely. We court sensitivity in order to enhance *tension on the move*. We respect tension, developing an intelligent relationship with it, because tension is intelligence. Working deeply reveals a primal unfettered tension. Individual tension opens up, inviting primal tension to come through.

An awareness of tensional quality is essential. There is a polarity between what happens in the body and our feeling of what happens. It is useful to realise that 'we don't know' exactly how much tension is needed to provide an intelligent balance. We don't need to know because, when given the opportunity, the organism is self-regulatory; *it knows*. When we go deeply with sensitivity, the older intelligence will reorganise itself and inform us of the requirements.

'It would seem therefore that the capacity for perfect doing is present in every man but must remain latent when conscious control is operative. The conscious is therefore a hindrance' (Feldenkrais 1949). His inference is not to abandon or ignore consciousness, but relates to how we use it. Tension responds to our consciousness of consciousness and its tendency to interfere, or not.

Thinking is tension because it involves activity; the gentlest of realisations arises from a culture of tension. It takes tension to register sensation because sensory nerves must act to convey information. No matter how receptive we may become, or to whatever extent we may not *do*, tension is there, like a creature, awaiting further instructions from the habitual mind. Tension is ever-present. Others may see it, point it out and help us to work with it, but it is our experience. Only we can fine tune, embrace and negotiate with our tension and its ever-changing nature. We are the final authority. Tension is our guide and mentor and only asks to be listened to. The power of deep primal tension on the move *reveals itself* when we do the work. Tension is negative when it grips, holds and inhibits any action but positive when it sustains, supports, and furthers appropriate action. *There is knowledge of expansion – but no knowledge in expansion. Expansion is an organic property expressing itself because this is what it does.*

Common Denominators

Common denominators

Observing a group, you see living, feeling organisms that share common denominators. Each member has contact with the ground, has the same skeletal arrangement and breathes. Each individual brings the basic physiological properties of the species into the practice. An individual sense of physiology is the route to, and interpreter of, primal presence. Common original physiology is acknowledged by individual consciousness. We can return to an original state as our starting point.

All practices, whether focused on postures, flow, spontaneous movement or the breath, are *physiological*. Deepening the physiological sense deepens practice. Regular application of a chosen style of working may have a deepening effect, but focusing on depth as the primary aspect enhances all work and provides a practice in itself. Depth work heightens the potential of all other practices.

We all take into practice the fact that we have:

- come from an aquatic environment,
- unfolded from land,
- contact with the earth,
- unfolded as embryos,
- a centre of gravity,
- a perpendicular gravity line around which all movement takes place,
- a spine,
- a thoracic cage,
- deep spinal diaphragmatic attachments,
- long bones feeding back through pelvic and shoulder girdles into the spine,
- an exhalation and inhalation,
- a substantial fluid content,
- skin and its connection to a central nervous system,
- sensory nerves,
- soft tissue that responds to gravity,
- a combination of acquired and inherent tension,
- the faculties of attention and awareness,
- a personal history,
- a tendency towards self-interference,
- deep involuntary movement that spreads throughout the body,
- the possibility of deepening and reinforcing the body-mind relationship,
- an unknown element that lies beneath practice,
- a relationship to time.

The Involuntary Unknown

Involuntary activity is a 'collective experience'. We get out of the way for something deeper to emerge. Our ways in (to the body-mind) may vary but the 'way out' tends to follow a basic organic tendency to unfold. Involuntary movement may be hidden from awareness and we may impose on it by using insensitive practices, but in essence involuntary movement cannot be customised or habituated. Involuntary movement provides the font from which we spring into voluntary movement and into ourselves.

Involuntary activity may be a familiar experience. The simple involuntary elongation of the spine may be known to many practitioners. At some point in time it may have been an unknown experience that became known as it surfaced, organic properties remain unknown until revealed. We can access detailed information regarding involuntary movement and know it in our heads, but to *feel* the deep movements of the spine and breath and the deep fluid of the body is to know by direct experience. The experience is ongoing, ever-changing and is not fixed by sensory imagination.

We are not innocent; perhaps naive in some respects but far from innocent. We know, expect, want and anticipate as we go into the primal areas of the body. But innocence in practice lies beneath the surface, and the deeper we go the more innocent we are invited to become. The deep body has a basic instinct for survival and an innate need to express itself; all else is superfluous in comparison. When we are simple, free from techniques and ideas, the innocence of the body arises and draws us into a way of moving that is un-held, powerful and transformational. Innocence implies pure, unpolluted, an authentic state free from the restrictions of systems. When we release the brakes of our conditioning we *all tend to move in the same way — the essential common denominator is our primality.*

A Common Pace

Although we may function at an individual pace, going inward is generally more productive when we give the tissues time to open up. As far as we can tell, life on this planet unfolded in its own organic time. Cells and systems must have needed time for cultivation and integration. Organic and mechanical development would have lain fallow between periods of intense activity. Slowing down in order to *feel more* enhances progress. When we wait a little, the deeper movements are given the time they might need to come towards us. Moving in too quickly can block a primal activity that might be on the way out. The natural behaviour of the organism arises when we remember to wait.

Waiting:

- calms the thinking mind, opens the sensory mind and enhances the assessment of moment-to-moment tension,

- enables the spine and the breath to augment each other — the natural pauses following the exhalations have time to read blood chemistry — the inhalations arrive as the spine is opening,

- gives time for the spine to maximise its intelligence and reveal itself,

- gives time for the articulations to open,

- gives time for the deep body and the skin to work together,

- enhances the action of the posterior fibres of the diaphragm in opening the front of the spine and move the body as a whole,

- gives a clearer perception of the relationship between the spine and the limbs, between the limbs and each other, and between the spinal curves and the individual vertebrae,

- enhances the pull of the earth and encourages the mechanical feel to develop into a softer feel,

- encourages the body to pull itself together spontaneously,

- gives an opportunity for the impediments of habit and conditioning to let go.

There is not one negative factor that arises from waiting, other than impatience. There is nothing to lose and much to gain by waiting for *the action to arrive.* Patience brings common denominators together in a synthesis of physiological expression.

When you have less time, or for just fun, you can engage with a faster practice and feel the benefits of the slower work come from a deeper and more grounded place. There is no need to give up your chosen practice. If there is a transition, then it will come by itself. The point is to be aware that there is an underlying practice that augments the primal expression of the body. You can move between practices, and alternate or incorporate them as the spirit moves you. If your body gravitates towards a quieter, deeper, more revealing experience, it would be common sense to oblige.

The most obvious common thread running through all practices is the fact that *we practice*, and that as practitioners we are influenced by the conditioning that accompanies personal history. The physiology of practice provides common ground between us, but so do the impediments that arise along the way. The realisation that beneath familiar aspects we can find an authentic way of being is enlightening. The discovery that authenticity arises from an original state common to all is even more enlightening.

Integration, Expression and Freedom

Integration

> *Primal movement is integrative and expressive.*
> *Integration and expression are linked. The deep natural*
> *movements of the spine move out to the periphery and*
> *all parts express a unified action True integration means*
> *that every vertebra and every peripheral articulation*
> *express their inter-relationship and their connection to*
> *the whole.*

We begin life with the potential for becoming integrated organisms (all else equal). This potential is challenged by various influences, some of which may involve imbalances at birth, but the majority of causes arise through and beyond the growing years.

Differentiation is the essential feature of embryonic development, a movement of the expression of life. Differentiation, which implies opening out into more functions and components than you started with, can also be seen as an expansion. Our tissues and systems have differentiated from a common source and retain an inherent relationship. For example, following implantation, a fertilised ovum soon differentiates into three primary germ layers (ectoderm, endoderm and mesoderm) from which all tissues and organs of the body develop.

Division, on the other hand, implies a separation of parts. When we divide, either anatomically, during practice or both, we overlook the natural tendency for the body to move as a whole. Division is divisive. Although individual muscles and muscle groups have specific functions, and at times may be seen or felt to work independently, they remain in relationship

through their mutual origin. Everything has the potential to 'pull together'. Mapping anatomical detail informs our understanding of relationship and depth, but it is more helpful to focus on basic aspects rather than be distracted by details that might overload our imagination as we work.

We are not trying to fit the experience into the anatomy but are inviting the anatomy into the experience. Although this distinction is not always clear, we should be aware that identifying an experience anatomically is more productive than practising from an idea of the anatomy.

The relevant anatomy concerns what we can, or may potentially feel. If you are levering your leg against your pelvis and spine you need to be aware of the anatomy to appreciate the risk. If you are feeding your arm back into your ribs, visualising the anatomy gives mechanical credence to the procedure, and the experience of your spine is enhanced by the visualisation.

The deeper we go into ourselves, the deeper the focus, the more integrated the approach to integration. A background in yoga and osteopathy has stimulated a personal sensory interest in articulations and their relationship, but you can enter the system from any perspective. All anatomical perspectives tend to lead in the same direction, with the same fluid result.

Rolfing, Structural Integration and similar approaches focus predominately on fascia as an integrative factor. Classic osteopathy integrates through the articulations. Anatomically, it is all connected. You cannot work with one aspect without influencing the others. Yoga, Feldenkrais, Alexander Technique, Continuum and other approaches tend to integrate the body, the mind and body, and the individual with the environment. We can always come across an aspect of ourselves that can reintegrate with the whole.

Not only can we work with every part of the body, for example, the thorax, hips, spine, shoulder and so on, but we can also focus on the various tissues. We can sense bone, soft tissue, articulations and skin. Integration involves blending the deepest areas with each other and with the outer layers. Skin on the outside and bone on the inside can occupy perception simultaneously.

Strength is found in integration. The inherent power of the organism is not realised by exercising specific muscle groups although this may be beneficial. Power comes from awakening a deep activity that fosters an integrated relationship between parts.

Freedom, Resistance and Articular Coherence

Personal conditioning may inhibit freedom of movement. The deep body submerges beneath layers of external influences; some may be necessary, and some counter personal growth and expression. Below the constraints of social, cultural and familial influence lies an inherent freedom that can be encouraged to surface, and to do so in a way that enhances other aspects of existence.

Any principles relating to physiological freedom are useful but also limited because understanding freedom necessitates direct experience. You can experience freedom without knowing the principles and you may understand the principles but lack the freedom. In practice, we can free ourselves from the idea of principles and *feel them*. Combining an understanding of basic principles with sensory experience is useful on all levels.

If we work within our limits and don't prioritise range of movement, we are free to work deeply without external resistance. When the body meets resistance it loses the freedom to reintegrate and express itself. Stretching does not guarantee integration or inner strength. Total freedom at all joints may be unrealistic, while a good measure of freedom accompanied by an integrated relationship between articulations as an outcome is more intelligent. There is a sense of freedom that considers range of movement secondary to a sense of a powerful expansion emanating from within *that may appear to inhibit freedom.*

Mabel Todd writes:

In the new born infant, the spine is straight and very flexible, with all joints movable. The first muscles to attain power are those of the lumbar spine and the pelvis, which the baby uses even before birth, squirming about, moving and straightening the lower back, drawing up the knees, and throwing them out in the 'kick' familiar to all mothers. For some time after birth the active muscles are those which are centring, that is holding the parts back against the spine, which is their centre of support. Thus, arms and legs tend to be held close to the body, as before birth. Later, when the more expansive movements take place, the ex-centring muscles, that is, those pulling weights away from the centres of support, become active in response to self-determined impulses and desires for movement (Todd 1937).

We may need to sacrifice range of movement for the deep tension of integration, which may hold us back initially but will also open the body in an integrated way. Freedom at the hips in a forward bend may be accompanied by restricted sections of the spine that impair a working relationship between the pelvis and shoulders.

When freedom is lost in one area it is usually compensated for in another area. For example, a sacroiliac joint will bear the brunt of its more constricted counterpart on the other side. An intelligent approach would be to hold back on both sides and work from within the pelvis as a whole without imposing the mechanical stress brought on by stretching the back of the pelvis and lumbar spine.

'Each articulatory unit expresses the dynamic forces of the body as a whole at any given time reacting to the several articular activities and the environment in which the body is at the moment' (Littlejohn 1898).

Freedom at some joints does not imply elasticity. Elasticity is a quality that enables tissue to open, release, return to its previous length and *meld* with the rest of the system. A relatively flexible body may not have a good quality of elasticity. Someone may have flexible hips and shoulders but sleepy tissue. Sleepy tissue implies dullness and a lack of responsive sensitivity. Range of movement may be predominately articular in nature but the tissues surrounding the bones may lack a feeling of aliveness. This may be due to overstretching, hereditary factors or a spine that is not communicating with the outer layers.

Elasticity is a textural quality that you can feel in the life and pulsation of the tissue. Freedom in the hips may give the impression of flexibility. Placing the chest upon fully extended knees may come easily but this is not an indication of an elastically responsive spine.

Freedom comes from disengaging the large outer layers and exploring the deeper layers around and between the spinal vertebrae. Treat your external tissue as a primal creature wrapped around your bones awaiting your sensitivity, interest and guidance. Once the inner body has engaged, the external tissues can take part and reorganise in relation to deeper tissue and articular activity.

There are two fundamental sensations of resistance: resistance of the large external muscles which may be felt as tightness or stiffness, and resistance of the deep body opening itself out to the surface, which is felt as an expansion from within. This overall expansion signifies deep and integrated articular coherence. The articulations actively respond to each other throughout the entire system. The freedom is in the rhythm between the vertebrae from tail to cranium and spreading out into the rest of the body. Freedom is found in rhythmic dynamic expression.

Continually returning to the centre and moving from there holds us back; it feels as if we are working against resistance. This is the resistance of integration; the articulations open up spatially and share their resistance throughout. Integration does not imply a completely free range at all movable joints; rather, it implies the quality of inter-joint relationship and comes from the combined interspatial element within each joint.

Although joint structure and function differs – synovial joints are cavities, disc joints are cartilaginous, cranial joints are fibrous, unfolding from within provides a tension that is picked up and integrated throughout all categories. Joints are supported externally and internally. We can approach them from the outside and from the inside. They are generally packed with cartilage and fluid but must also maintain inner and outer tension by connective tissue engagement. The term, 'freely movable joint' is relative.

We like to *feel open* in the body unless openness poses a threat to security. A young woman was emotionally bound in her shoulders to the extent that she could not raise her arms above shoulder height without bursting into tears. There are other more extreme examples, but suffice to say there may be substantial investment in 'containing oneself', and opening should take the time

that it needs. Even more reason to centre and ground oneself, and move from there.

Mechanical Stress

Intelligent work acknowledges a balance of natural stresses that play through the body at all times. These stresses can be exaggerated or balanced by practice. A great deal of negative stress occurs beneath our awareness and leads to problems if continually exaggerated.

All mechanical stress involves variations of pressure or tension, i.e. parts of the body being either pushed together or pulled apart. Gravity over time can be the main offender. X-rays and scans of spines demonstrate the effects of gravity on many people, some of whom are otherwise relatively healthy. The spine may wear away quite comfortably before pain and dysfunction set in. Teachers are not exempt from disc injury or sacroiliac strain. I know several yoga teachers with hip replacements. They might have required surgery at some point with or without yoga, and it is possible that the onset of pain and disability was delayed by their practices. The point is that there are no guarantees. Working from within to open the joints evenly, and sensing the articulations as a system in their own right, would appear to be an intelligent way to proceed. Range of movement should come by itself and not be the primary focus. Those with 'new hips' continue to practice, and do so with continued benefit, but with the understanding that containment remains an important aspect of their approach. Figures 6.1 through to 6.4A depict the deformation of spinal discs as a consequence of mechanical stresses, which if prolonged or habituated may incur permanent damage and impact on surrounding tissues and bone. Further to this, disturbance or dysfunction between any two or more vertebrae, disrupts the fluidity of the spine and its integration with the rest of the body in practice.

Mabel Todd, in her classic book *The Thinking Body*, identifies five mechanical stresses:

- Compression stress is the most prevalent stress, pushes joints together, and is easily exaggerated.

- Tensile stress is the opposite of compression, as it involves parts pulling away from each other.

- Torsion stress twists parts of the body around its long axis and involves alternate compression and tensile stress.

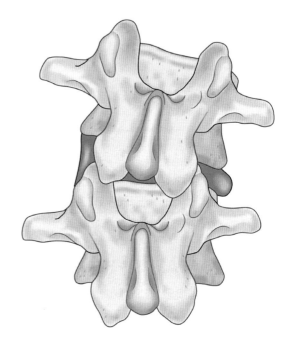

Figure 6.2

Stress – side-bending lumbar spine, tensile and compression stress.

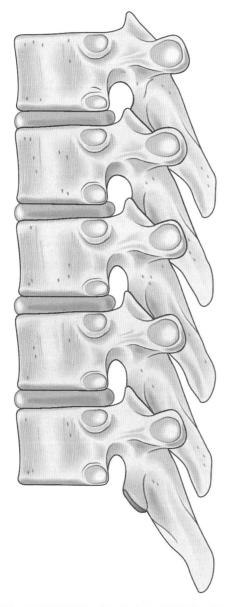

Figure 6.1

Compression stress of the dorsal spine.

- Shear is a force directed at an angle to the axis, one part slides on another with potential disturbance of the axis.

- Bending stress combines tension and compression, curves the axis of the spine and potentially weakens strength and support.

We might have a clearer sense of these stresses as our sensitivity increases. Common examples of overstressing joints and tissues in practice are:

- Sustaining a forward bending of the spine and locking several vertebrae by soft tissue tension. Bending the spine for any length of time inhibits spinal fluidity. Bending is beneficial when combined with articular and respiratory rhythm and centring the thigh and arm bones. The bend however will come by itself and when the body is rhythmically awake will tend to unbend itself.

- Backward bending may create shearing stress between the fifth lumbar vertebra and the sacrum.

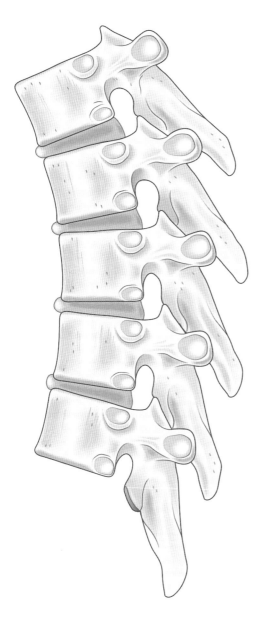

Figure 6.3A

Stress – forward-bending dorsal spine.

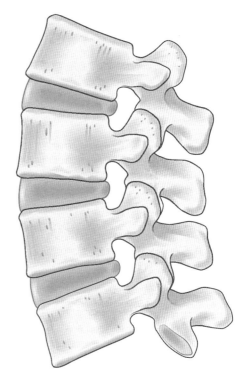

Figure 6.3B

Stress – backward-bending lumbar spine.

The bending should be secondary to articular spacing and the support of the diaphragm, abdominal muscles and the long bones – in other words, the entire body works to negate the stress. When we are in the rhythmic fluid stage, the softening of tissues will render mechanical precautions less necessary. We feel impending stress more clearly and avoid it. But precautions should be taken.

- Twisting a sleepy spine exaggerates torsional stress. The discs should be open and soft to maximise their potential. Rotation is a common osteopathic procedure for 'locking down' the spine to prepare for an adjustment. We should not invite locking, as it inhibits fluidity and deep respiration. Torsion is positive when it happens spontaneously as a consequence of the action at the front of the spine.

- Compression of the medial aspect of the knee in standing work, or overstretching the knees in knee folded attitudes. In effect, knees remain healthy when they are rhythmically responsive to the breath and spine.

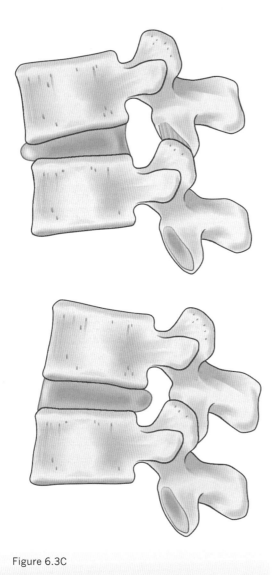

Figure 6.3C

Stress – shearing stress lumbar spine.

the upward thrust from the ground and a deeply active spine. The upper body complex, the spine and lower body share an original evolutionary source and comprise an *articulatory system.*

When the focus is on small movements, such as those stimulated by breathing and attention given to containing the spine, the potential for minimising stress is enhanced. Intervertebral rhythm is an indication that the spine and peripheral joints and tissues are stress free.

When the body expresses itself from deeply within, the mechanical stresses tend to work for and not against us. As compression and tensile stress adjust to each other, the effects of torsion, shearing and bending are taken up by all the articulations as they open and communicate with each other. Each position should spread throughout the entire body and involve all tissues and articulations.

Teachers are not exempt from wear and tear. Arthritic hips and knees, degenerative discs and sacroiliac dysfunction are not uncommon. Many bodies are not suitable for certain positions. A pre-posture approach maximises benefits and avoiding strain. The posture in mind may even feel unwanted when the body finds its own expression. This involves engaging the muscles closest to the spine, centring your bones and opening your inner articular space. Tension in the outer layers may be the consequence of mechanical incoherence on the inside.

There are many possibilities that may detract from safe and intelligent practice. There is not the space here to examine all the potential mechanical risks in various positions and how to modify them. An across-the-board approach would be to strengthen and open the body from inside out. This is achievable by gravity work that encourages the upward thrust of the ground to open the articulations, by centring the long bones, and by working with the central mechanism to bring the body back to its softer, more fluid organic qualities. Mechanical stress is negated when the organism is in ascendance – but we must work for this. Figure 6.4b shows the intervertebral spaces without discs. This depiction is synonymous with the feeling of spinal spatiality and freedom.

Everyone has a degree of scoliosis, a sideways curvature of the spine, a weak and strong side. These imbalances vary in shape between individuals, and come with

Overstretching generally creates repeated tensile stress and can lead to problems. All weight-bearing joints are subject to pressure and distraction. Pressure on one side of a joint is balanced by compensatory distraction on the other side. Compression and tensile stress are *axial*, as they run through the long axis of the body. Non-weight-bearing joints such as those of the shoulder and arm complex and the jaw also respond to

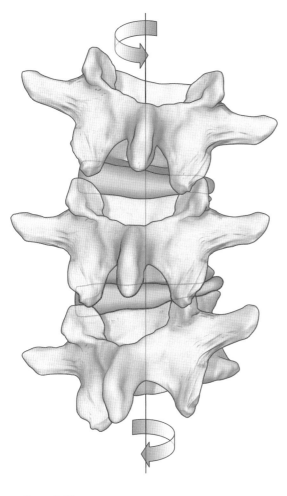

Figure 6.4A

Partial common scoliosis.

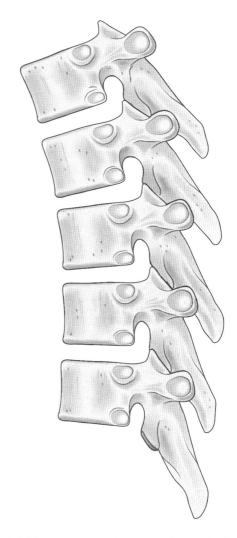

Figure 6.4B

Inter-vertebral spaces.

degrees of rotation either towards or away from the convexity of the curve. Many imbalances are so slight they are hardly noticeable, but they exist and involve excessive compression and tensile stress on each side of the spine. We all have a pull towards one side or the other. Everyone, in practice, has a 'good' or 'bad' side. The way forward is to work on the weak side, by creating more space in the foot, leg, drawing back more and working the diaphragm and pelvic floor on that side. Trying to bend the spine away from the convexity 'to straighten it' can potentially weaken the curves. We can approach it from the front of the spine and limb on the weak side.

There are few perfect spines, as thoracic or lumbar areas may be excessively curved one way or the other, and the sacrum may be off centre and so on. Treatment aside, we work with what we have. When working with the spine as a whole, from the ground, with the long bones of the limbs, the deep central muscles and with the breath, we can encourage a stronger and more integrated vertebral column from within. The spine will often reorganise itself as it regains its deep power.

Expression

Freedom for the organism to express itself is not the freedom of disengagement, floppiness or joint laxity. The organism expresses itself freely and actively by engaging articular coherence. As we grow embryonically, we unfold from a central source, and engagement spreads out into the soles of the feet, the toes, fingers and palms. Our primary movement patterns involved *pushing out against our own resistance*. This expressive activity involves articulations, muscle, connective tissue and bone. We segment, pushing outwards from a centre that holds its periphery close. We open up against an inherent tension that will eventually provide the underpinning for the articular coherence and engagement needed for support and movement under gravitational pull.

To re-experience this primal expression:

- open the areas closest to the ground, e.g. the arches of your feet and your ankles when standing, the elbows and wrists in downward positions,

- keep the long bones of your limbs close to the central axis of the spine, i.e. feed them back in order to minimise pulls on your deep body and maximise spinal release and action,

- keep your knees and elbows bent to enable a conversant relationship between all articulations feeding back into the spine,

- observe the gravitational elements at all times, using your body weight, if necessary, in any position by consolidating your contact points,

- keep the attention on your spine and its relationship to the rest of your body,

- when in doubt, back off, take out the tension and renegotiate,

- *keep coming back to your centre, the space and the deep expression of inter-articular activity.*

- re-activate the hands and feet.

When we work from the inside out, the tissues are countered from within. True freedom is found by releasing the potential of your deep body so that it can act! Open your outer by activating your inner.

A Suitable Arrangement

The skeletal framework's design is telling: we can see and sense its shape. There is a small base, and long lower limbs pointing towards and away from the ground and attaching to the spine through the pelvis. Long upper limbs moving towards and away from their surrounding space are loosely attached to the thorax and spine through the shoulder girdle. One continuous *inner space* is made up of a thoracic, abdominal and pelvic cavity. There is an axial spine made up of four opposing curves to support weight, and from which all movement is directed from and to. This entire bony arrangement is representative of a mechanism that has unfolded from the ground.

The inspiring pioneer of osteopathy, John Martin Littlejohn, had this to say about the bones:

The bones are the primary objective because they form the fundamental framework to which all structures are attached. In the spine the attention should not be given to the muscles along it but to the fibro-cartilaginous discs through appropriate movement. The muscles do perform the function of mobility in the spine while the fibro-cartilage resists up to a point to maintain the integrity of each segment and prevent each segment functioning by itself. ... All the functional and supportive structures of the body have their terminal point in a bone. Leverage, muscular and ligamentous activity and fascial conciliation depend on the bone as it moves in an articular unit with a definitive system of activity (Littlejohn 1898).

Visualise the shape of your bones and their relationship. They provide the supportive architecture enabling the integrated emergence of primal movement.

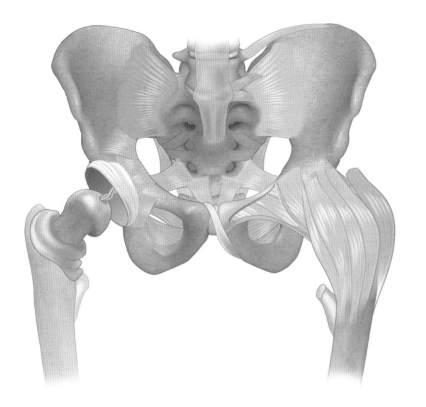

Figure 6.5

Organs of separation – hip.

Organs of Space

The articulations are organs of movement, separation and perception. We can feel them open. The word *open* has numerous definitions, but those most applicable to our work include unbounded, unobstructed, revealed, made known, unfold the sense of and enlighten. Opening the articular system can be a profound experience.

Each joint is an organ in its own right integrating with the whole. We can sense our articulations as organs of movement, but just as relevant, is the sense of inter-articular space and engagement. Given that joints are packed with tissue, fluid, cartilage and/or fibrous material, space in a joint applies to the space between bones. You can feel inter-articular space because the tissue within and around the joints is richly endowed with sensory nerves. When you feel into your hip, shoulder, ankle or spine, you are receiving information from soft, sensitive, spacious and intelligent organs. Articulations pulsate, interact, move and rhythmically open and close. Articulations express the forces that

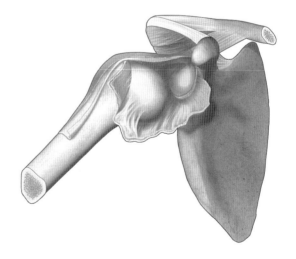

Figure 6.6

Organs of separation – shoulder.

run through the body and are an integral part of our expressive nature.

The Decisive Organ

Muscles are organs of expression, and perform our voluntary movements. They hold us, grip and release our bones, our joints, our breath and our feelings. Tension, whether superfluous, deep, transient, well-established, postural or emotional lies in muscle tissue. Muscles are the first line of defence under all circumstances. They may be tense and reactive or soft, yielding and responsive.

By virtue of their natural reflexes and underlying tone, muscles are never free from tension. It's a matter of degree. Ideally, we use the minimum amount of tension to work in postures but certain areas may need sustained work to keep the space, such as the ankles and arches of the feet in standing. We need to work the central muscles to realise softness and fluidity throughout the body a whole.

We tend to present ourselves to the world through external muscles. They express our persona. 'Here I am' presentations are delivered through the external layers. Deeper layers may need release and action but the outer tend to take the rein, lest we lose our guard. Most obviously, the facial tissues display the persona we wish to convey. We may repress expression anywhere, close to the spine, the thoracic and pelvic diaphragms, the arches of the feet, the long thigh muscles or anywhere. Our sense of self is coloured by muscle sense.

Individual muscle activity is reflected in their shape and size. Muscles may be long, broad, thick, fine, short or small, but they can all function as one extensive organ. Muscles are neurologically connected through the spinal cord, mechanically connected through fascia and also connected through a fluid dynamic. Identifying specific muscle action may be useful to a point, but once identified it is more helpful to sense muscle as an organic sleeve encompassing the bones. We may work with a specific area but feeling its connection to the rest of the system is essential for integration. For example, the thoracic diaphragm may deepen its activity but its connection to the spine, shoulder

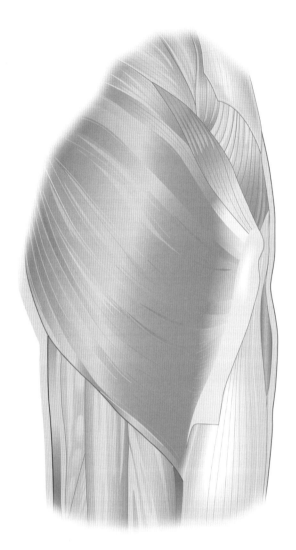

Figure 6.7A

Muscle – as an organ.

and pelvic girdle muscles provides an upper and lower body response.

We can perceive muscle as one complete organ providing a background or foreground to our general experience. Working with muscle tension and its conditioning is an essential feature in practice. Muscle activity and tone are barometers of how we are feeling and how we should proceed in practice. How far in we go, and in what way we do so depends upon our negotiation with

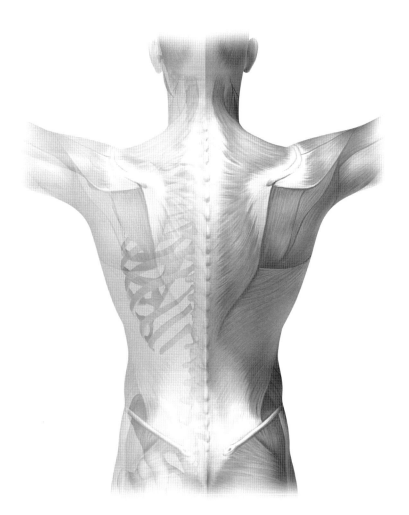

Figure 6.7B

Muscle – sleeving bone.

muscle tension. We may exaggerate or release our sense of self through the muscles, depending upon a requirement usually revealed by the deep body. Real change comes from the perception of all muscles as one entire organ with an inner and outer element. Figure 6.7A gives a sense of the organic power of muscle tissue and as an organ in its own right. Figure 6.7B gives a sense of muscle sleeving bone.

The Fascial Connector

The first thing to understand about anatomy is that everything is connected. It's not surprising that connective tissue holds such interest in the body-mind world. Muscles are our executive organs but fascia is the organ of connectivity and integration, and has been an essential factor in our development. 'In the embryo, it is largely the proliferation of connective tissue structures which serves as a blueprint for the growth of the rest of the body's bulk' (Juhan 1987).

The relevance of fascia in body work was highlighted by Rolfing and Structural Integration practitioners. Their research continues to support their work and influence fitness and movement specialists and yoga teachers. Research and recent literature on fascia is almost as extensive as the fascia itself. Fascia is currently dominating the world of body-work and it is easy to see why. It is the primary connective tissue and connects each and every part of the organism. Fascia plays

an essential mechanical role and is involved in neurological and chemical activity. Due to its texture and
all-pervasive nature, fascia can be seen as an organism
within the organism. Figures 6.8A and 6.8B show the
gross connection of fascia and muscle through the leg.

'No longer perceived as a passive network of connective tissue, fascia is seen as an essential agent in
movement and support and an integral component of
articular and muscular activity. Fascia is invested in and
encapsulates virtually all tissues in the body' (Langevin
& Huijing 2009).

Many discoveries regarding fascial activity concern
its chemistry and finer mechanical details. We sense
the gross aspects of fascia, although these have subtle
elements. Fascia draws us together, opens us out, and also
pulsates. We can feel the fascial body draw itself together
and also feel the lightest local activity. When you feel
your body pulling together and opening out, it is through
the agency of fascia working in concert with muscles and
bones to open and connect your articulations. Fascia enables you to engage your ankles and feel the action in your
pelvis, spine, shoulder jaw and cranium.

B.K.S Iyengar continuously referred to the skin as an
active agent. He was feeling his skin, but this feeling
must have included the superficial fascia which connects deeply into the spine.

Evidence suggests that fascia has a contractile capabil-
ity (Staubesand & Li 1996). Fascia has a role in opening
and closing articulations, in drawing the bones towards
and away from the centre. The relevance of fascia is not
a recent discovery. The founder of osteopathy, Andrew
Taylor Still, wrote in 1902:

I know of no part of the body that equals the fascia as a
hunting ground. Still one part is just as great as any other in
its place. No part can be dispensed with. ... A knowledge of
the universal extent of the fascia is imperative and is one of
the greatest aids to the person who seeks the causes of disease
(Still 1902).

Fascia works in conjunction with muscle, articulations,
bone and fluid. Fascial (myofascial) integration implies
the entire network moving as one supportive and expansive organ. According to the research of Robert Schleip
who has conducted extensive research on fascia, there
are ten times more sensory receptors in fascial tissues
than there are in muscles (Shleip 2012).

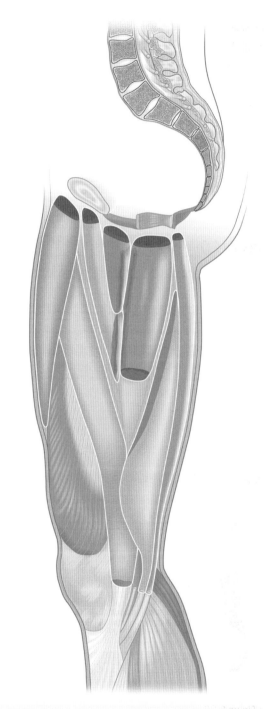

Figure 6.8A

Fascia – inner thigh.

Give your weight to the ground and move away from the ground. Move deeply inside yourself – move from the spine – give your long bones back to the centre – give your spine back to itself – consolidate your base by opening the joints closest to the ground. Unfold actively from deeply within yourself – the postures are secondary to the process of unfolding and centring. Feel the resistance as you work, as the bones push out against the restraining activity of the myofascial organ.

Yoga and Osteopathy

Several parallels can be found between osteopathy and yoga, not least of all a primary interest in

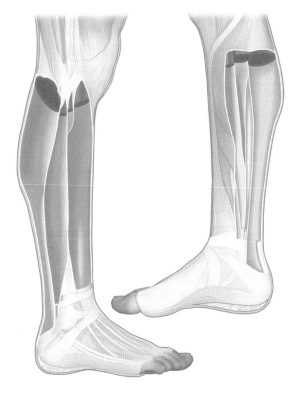

Figure 6.8B

Fascia – lower leg.

mechanical balance. Yoga teachers and osteopaths (and others in similar fields) share an interest in freeing the body from restrictions and fixations, and integrating the parts with the whole. As teachers, we work with spinal mechanics, connective tissue, articular integration and other aspect of physiology normally associated with osteopathy and body work. We may do this without realising the full integrative effectiveness of our approach.

Osteopathic principles and practice are particularly concerned with the deep body, and the primal movements of the spine. Osteopathic clients can *unwind* in a deep and spontaneous spiral as the spine finds its freedom and deeper nature. This action is common in our practice when we have relinquished the surface tension, deepened the focus, and moved aside for the spine to reveal itself.

Osteopathy recognises the importance of the intersegmental muscles of the spine column. These words from *The Physiological Basis of Osteopathic Medicine* highlight this recognition: 'Clearly these small muscles and the finely tuned motions they control are crucial factors in chronic musculoskeletal disorders and the associated cost of a patient's posture and locomotion'. In our practice, we engage with these muscles continually, as they represent the essence of core activity and potential for primal movement.

From the Postgraduate Institute of Osteopathic Medicine and Surgery:

Inter-segmental mobility is very finely tuned by the small and easily forgotten muscles that run from segment to segment. Their critical role is not always appreciated in considerations of long range degenerative changes. We can see that the large muscles, for example, the erector spinal group, initiate large movements, but what mediates the translation of forces from one segment to the next? The inter-segmental muscles are the conditioning agents and if their function is disturbed the result may be a change in the tracking characteristics at that particular segmental junction, which in time will show impaired function. We begin to see the constant drain that this causes, the excessive cost of normal daily activities (Postgraduate Institute 1970).

This osteopathic observation confirms the relevance of 'getting into the spine', and staying there, as and

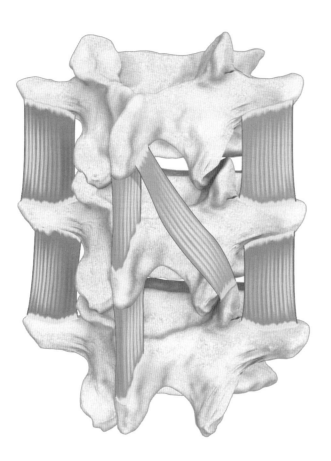

Figure 6.9A

Intervertebral muscles.

when necessary. Figures 6.9A and 6.9B depict the anatomical relevance of the smaller spinal muscles. They present as an integral 'part of the spine'.

Yoga teachers may use their hands to promote feeling in a certain area, hold people back, or reorganise bones. Yoga adjustments are popular and beneficial. Some of the adjustments I have received from the well-informed hands of teachers have in their own way been particularly effective. Our objective is to impart feeling, space and direction as opposed to effecting pain relief, although pain resolution may happen spontaneously.

In osteopathic and yoga practice you *think and feel* into the body. An osteopathic approach known as *articulation* gives the long bones back to the centre and rhythmically unwinds and integrates the body using the limbs as sensitive levers to integrate the girdles, the various areas of the spine and the individual vertebrae. We can feel these connections for ourselves. For example,

feeding our femur into the lumbar area gives an active response through the entire length of the spine, up into the shoulder, neck and jaw. Changing the angle of the limb influences different parts of the spine.

We can *feel* the spinal rhythm through the limbs, and sense the spinal articulations opening up in response to the active centring of the long bones. We can also observe the effect in the opposite direction, from the spine to the limbs. For example, opening up the thoracic spine creates more space and action through the shoulder girdle, elbow, wrists and activates the hands and fingers.

The osteopath uses his manual skills, understanding of mechanics, and sensory perception when treating another person. We penetrate our own body using our own sensory perception, and depending on the messages we receive, make the appropriate adjustments. Both practices require undisturbed attention and are based on *what is felt*.

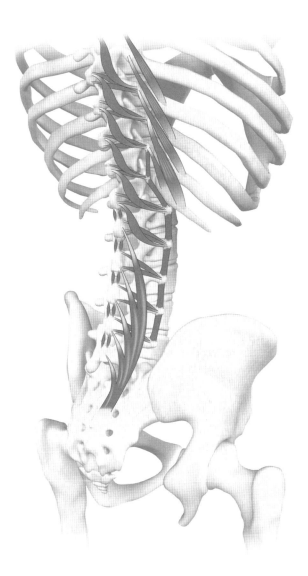

Figure 6.9B

Small spinal muscles throughout.

The common ground between yoga and osteopathy is the focus on physiological integration. The founder of osteopathy, A.T. Still, suggested that the real work was to adjust someone to their total environment by considering all aspects of the human being. As yoga teachers, we point students in a direction that enables them to undertake this consideration for themselves.

Yoga teachers and osteopaths can learn from each other. In all aspects of our work, we come back to the fact that the body is an expressively responsive organ, constantly adjusting to the stresses that play through it, not least of which is 'how we are'. That is, our bodies have to deal with us. Maximising the practical implications of this realisation involves trusting our perceptual instincts, facilitating exploration and getting out of our way at the right time.

We gather in – push out – differentiate – integrate unfold – sometimes in the same moment. Returning to an original state is not a passive affair; it is not relaxation, although relaxation may be a requirement. An original state awakens a deeply active strength. As we progressed from early beginnings, we lifted ourselves up and extended outwards. We achieved this through direct purchase on the earth and from a strong and active centre. In practice, we can begin again, unfolding into life from a grounded and centred personal resolve. At this point of integration, one can return to a primal fluid state.

When the body undoes and unwinds there are no mechanical laws to follow. Apart from occasionally returning to the base of support and re-gravitating, there are no sophisticated rules of procedure. We start with mechanics, move into organics and graduate to a fluid state. We discover that fluid is a connective tissue; it is everywhere, reducing differentiation and division into a wave-like mobility free from mechanical stress and the ideas surrounding it.

Exploratory Tools

You

> *We could be physiological archaeologists, digging deeply into ourselves in order to reveal ancient properties that lie within. The deeper we go the more refined the tools, lest we disturb the intelligence that lies beneath the soil of our conditioning.*

Working methods, however effective, pale in light of your own inquiry. You are the tool for deepening practice. You are on site experiencing your tensions, weaknesses, impediments and realisations. The most useful tools are within us. *You* are the working tool and the immediate recipient of your exploration.

Within the field of you (us) various components coalesce to produce a working approach. The tools for going deeply may not be unfamiliar, but have a deeper and possibly more intense application. They are mutually supportive and can be broadly divided into body tools and mind tools.

Positions, movements, gravity, and breathing provide the physical tools. Mind tools include interest and curiosity, essential thought, visualisation, imagination, sensory appreciation, exploration and an acknowledgement of polarity. In essence, physical tools are mind tools because their efficiency depends on how we use them. Inspiration is also a powerful tool,* but you can't *do* inspiration, it *arises*. Inspiration drives exploration and is a consequence of a deeper experience. We begin to see the possibilities as original movement emerges. Self-inspired, investigative practice produces profound results. The following tools relate to the mind and underpin everything else that we use. The mind is the director, at least initially.

*The word *tool* comes from the old English *tawian* meaning 'to prepare.'

Essential Thought

The mind is the primary tool. Sensory information is made conscious by the mind as it explores and receives sensation. Sensory experience is received: we don't *do* experience, experience *arrives* into conscious awareness. How we experience sensation determines how we respond and how we respond determines the quality of further experience.

To enter physical depth we pass through layers of mental activity that are irrelevant to the work at hand. The mind becomes attentively sharp, a refined tool with which to move through itself and through tense and sleepy tissue.

We start with a mind that is clear and focused in order to minimise interference that clouds sensory perception. Essential thought focuses directly on the necessary ingredients for a deeper experience. As thought opens up awareness, the mind registers ongoing sensations and describes them to itself. The language of feeling thoughts registers and describes sensation and opens the door to the deeper body experience.

Feeling thoughts may describe heaviness, tension, weakness, responsiveness, pleasure, lightness, fluidity and anatomy, and may be punctuated by insight.

The original body 'felt' and responded long before the development of thought. Feeling is primal, thought is not. Thought arose from consciousness and consciousness arose from the body. Feeling thoughts, along with stimulation from the environment, may have been a precursor to thinking, as our primal ancestors sought to interpret what they felt. The point is that thought is here, and we use it to engage with the body.

We are not deep in thought but think deeply in to the body. Essential thought receives information from and enters into the abdominal, thoracic and pelvic cavities, the articulations and tissues. We can think between and around bones, into muscle, fascia and fluid, as the mind penetrates the body's mechanical and organic patterning.

Thinking becomes redundant with the progression of deep spontaneous movement. As you move deeply into yourself, the more you think the less you feel, and the more you feel the less you need to think. Primal movement is beyond suggestion and interpretation but thrives on attention. In its purest sense attention is free from thought. Sensation may be initiated by thought feelings but sensation takes over. The old adage 'I think therefore I am' might be a start but is rendered superfluous as the deep body emerges.

Imagination and Visualisation

Thought invites imagination and visualisation. The imagining, visualising mind directs and redirects in response to returning sensory information. Visualising and imagining, linked to awareness, are needed for deeper investigation because the body's innermost areas take time to awaken, they are elusive. We use the mind to *target* the shape of the lumbar vertebrae and facet joints and the texture of the discs. We imagine their potential for original movement. We are *on site* and can continue from there to awaken sensitivity.

We can imagine and visualise all kinds of activity within the positions that we use. As the senses awaken, the use of imagery/visualisation becomes stronger, more meaningful, and takes us even more deeply. When imagination and visualisation meet physiology the results can be profound. The work of Alexander and Feldenkrais, therapeutic dance, cranial and energy work and many other modalities use and enhance our ability to visualise the nature of anatomical features and physiological activity.

Although we use imagination and visualisation to enhance our ability to *feel inside ourselves* (imagine or visualise the diaphragm spreading its wings), it is the depth reached that determines the realisation and refinement of the deep areas.

James Oschman writes: 'Our images shape our therapeutic successes because they can give rise to specific intentions. Intentions are not trivial, because they give rise to specific patterns of electrical and magnetic activity in the nervous system of the therapist that can spread through their body of the patient' (Oschman 2000). In our practice we are *therapist and patient combined*. Our intention is to sense and enhance our original, unconditioned spine and deep body; this is what we do!

There are subtle differences between imagining and visualising. Imagination forms a mental concept of something that is not present or not yet in the senses. Imagining is a useful precursor to sensations not yet available to consciousness. Imagination can also mean *to meditate on something*. The spinal curves, the front of the sacrum and the dome of the diaphragm may be brought into awareness through imagination. We might imagine a deep involuntary opening of the jaw, or a relationship between the deep arch of the foot and the shoulder. Imagining possibilities can bring them closer to a felt physical reality.

Visualisation may be defined as 'forming a mental vision, *image* or picture' of (something). This is where basic anatomy is useful. We are using creative visualisation when we create an *image* of an articulation or bone in our mind's eye and visualise it moving. We cannot visually see our diaphragm or the front of our spine but we can mentally and physically engage with them through visualisation.

'Ideokinesis', or the 'idea of movement', is an expression used by Lulu Sweigard, a student of Mabel Todd. Sweigard introduces this term in her book *Human Movement Potential* (Sweigard 1974). She promotes *ideokinetic facilitation* as a means for improving human performance. Her practical techniques employ visualisation and imagined movement to good effect. For example, imagining the pelvis as a concertina opening at the back and closing at the front provides a basis for enhancing its mechanical behaviour.

Imagination invites sensation and promotes action and is exclusively personal to the imaginer. Imagining the elongation of the spine produces sensations of your spine elongating, imagining the softening of the facial muscles softens the facial muscles, and so on. We have only one nervous system which, one way or another, connects thought, imagination, sensory appreciation and action throughout the entire body.

Sensory Inquiry

Physiologists identify direct sensory pathways that convey and register feeling coming from deep and superficial parts of the body. This enables us to engage and negotiate with sensations of strain, pull, effort, release, space, freedom and a collection of myriad sensory impressions emerging and deepening during practice. As soon as we *feel more*, we realise sensation as the ultimate tool and the key to a deeper expression. Whether we focus on the skin, the muscles, the spine or the organism as a whole, sensation is the way in.

Can you feel your skin as an organ of perception; can you feel it right now across you back, over your thighs, through the upper arms and around your thorax? Can you sense the roots of your diaphragm or internal intercostal muscles? How much of your body can you feel acting in concert with an exhalation? Can you sense the shape of your bones, or feel your articulations as organs of separation? How often do you feel yourself as a total, thinking, feeling, tensile, pulsating organism, breathing and responding to gravity?

We experience the consequence of sensory nervous activity but do not feel the nervous activity itself. We feel tension in the muscles or articulations opening inside us, but we don't feel the nervous activity that produces the sensations. We only feel the consequence of sensory nervous activity. The feelings come from the organs that nerves supply. We are aware of thoughts and feelings and actions but not aware of the nervous activity that produces them. We can only focus on the organs and their activity but not the nerves associated with them. Enhancing organic awareness (articulations, muscles, and bones are organs) enhances their nervous connections and sensitivity. We don't focus on the brain when we think but thinking enhances the brains capacity for thinking.

Physical feeling is generally categorised into proprioceptive, interoceptive and exteroceptive sensations. We work with all of them. Proprioceptive sensations inform us of position, articular sense of movement and muscle tension. The word proprioception, meaning sense of self, comes from the Latin *proprius*, meaning *one's own* or *individual*, followed by *perception*. Interoceptive sensations convey feelings coming from the tissues, such as subtle streaming, release and tension. Exteroceptive sensations are concerned with sight, hearing and so on. Personal experience is based on the direct perception of your self coming from your self.

We are told that sensory nerve endings (proprioceptors) in muscles, tendons and articulations convey information to the cerebral cortex and their efficiency determines sensitivity in practice. Recent studies suggest that the fascial network works with sensory nerves to deliver sensation more rapidly to awareness. The sensory system is sensitive to tension. Too much or not enough tension dulls sensitivity. Research shows that a typical nerve feeding a muscle has three times the amount of sensory fibres than it does motor fibres (Schleip 2012), confirming that sensory appreciation is the essential factor in nervous activity — we are indeed a response to our environment.

The literature on sensory distribution gives little, if any, information on how deeply we can feel. Sensory activity must take place at the deepest levels in order for us to be supported and move under gravitational pull. Personal inquiry suggests that we may feel the intersegmental spinal muscles, the posterior roots of the diaphragm and the deep iliopsoas. We certainly feel the central area as an entirety, the superficial tissue of the waist and belly, and the deeper tissue drawing, pumping and releasing as we work. It is apparent that through practice we can develop an ongoing, deeper and stronger sense, and therefore understanding, of the spine and deep respiratory muscles and their relationship.

With the evolutionary flowering of the nervous system, we have dispensed with the perception of well-established sensory pathways, which function autonomously beneath conscious awareness. A perception of basic reflex sensations feeding back into the spinal cord serves no purpose. But it is possible to retrace some of our steps and awaken feelings related to basic behaviour.

The following information is unhelpful because we cannot feel the actual pathway of nervous conduction. Unconscious perception, i.e. sensations that we are not meant to feel, *is primarily communicated via the dorsal and ventral spino-cerebellar nervous pathways to the cerebellum. Conscious perception of feeling is communicated by the posterior column medial lemniscus pathway to the cerebrum.* But it is useful to know that unconscious perceptions do not register as high up in the brain as conscious perceptions and the information supports the personal experience that *non-essential mental activity interferes with physical perception and sensitivity.*

A sense of self at any level is dependent upon sensory nerves providing substantial nervous activity and taking up a large percentage of the nervous system. Sensing deeply and directly into core tissues does not necessitate intricate neuromuscular re-education. We can return to a pre-sophisticated state where the 'fine differences' of musculoskeletal differentiation will take care of themselves as core activity begins to take centre stage.

When I invite deep rotation, a perception that combines relevant thought, imagination, visualisation, and sensory appreciation moves respectfully and inquisitively inwards. An intimate process occurs between my body and myself as I pass through the external tissue, assessing spinal tension and everything associated with it. If I get caught up by the *word* 'proprioception' I inhibit the feeling and quality of rotation. Labelling the physiology of feeling and the feeling itself are incompatible beyond a certain point. The sensation is more helpful than the label. Sensation in the present is *ours* and is an original sensation.

In passing through the outer body and cutting through the external patterns we can also cut through a detailed approach. Once thought, imagination and sensory inquiry have opened the door; you are there, within your deeper physiological reality.

Moshe Feldenkrais writes: 'I suggest, and I believe that I am right, that sensory stimuli are closer to our unconscious, subconscious, or autonomous functioning than to any of our conscious understanding. On the sensory level communication is more directly associated with the unconscious, and is therefore more effective and less disturbed than at the verbal level' (Feldenkrais 1995).

When we go back through the evolutionary stages of thought, imagination, conscious sensation, and the pure sensation that normally lies beneath the level of conscious registration, we arrive at an action stimulated by a primitive sensory system, and as it comes into consciousness, it more or less wipes the slate clean.

Krishnamurti felt that 'Speculation and imagination were the enemies of attention', and when you look at it in yourself he has a point because pure unadulterated attention has no content, images, ideas or plans. But, we have to start somewhere.

Deep Movement and Exploration

Exploration is the foundation of intimate inquiry. Guided by sensation, we can adjust, delve and combine small external movements with spontaneous deeper ones. We can change position, shift contact points and stimulate new areas of the depth body.

The inner body experience is so expansive and total that you cannot pin it down to one thing. It changes from moment to moment. Exploration may be instigated by us but happens naturally as the body takes us on its own journey. Exploration, part manipulated, part spontaneous, invites unwavering attention, it keeps us interested, moves us from place to place and back again, sometimes in the same moment. Exploration moves from recess to recess, articulation to articulation, tension to tension, wave to wave and pulsation to pulsation.

Exploration invites and follows an inner dance, the creativity of the practitioner negotiating with the creative inner expression of the body. We move into and through resistance, waiting for it to melt or change, or use it to open more space. Inner space is vast. Articulations and body cavities may feel ever deepening. There is an entire spine to explore, an ever-deepening pelvis, the spaces between the long bones, the fluid and respiratory waves, openings and gatherings. One may feel as if one moves from the deepest places beyond the boundaries of the skin.

We might assume that some areas or functions are unfeelable, but should not underestimate someone else's capacity to feel. If someone says they can sense their cuboid, then perhaps they can, or perhaps they have an awareness of the skin overlying the cuboid, or perhaps a strong visual image gives an impression of sensation. The crux is that one way or another it is in awareness.

Movement promotes sensation, and in a relative sense, there are no areas in the body that are immovable. A section of bone may be perceived by the pulsation of its surrounding tissue and fluid. A small articulation may begin to move with the inner dance of the whole skeleton.

As we drop descriptions, the sensory cortex sits back and *goes with the flow*. This aspect of deepening practice cannot be taught; in essence you cannot capture sensations. Sensation itself is movement, constantly changing as it interacts with its internal and external environment. Sensation defies technique but we can describe *frameworks of sensation*. Expanding, centring, pulsing and waving are movements providing sensory frameworks that can be imparted. Experience is free from technique. You cannot teach sensation but you can lead others towards finding it.

Relationship and Polarity

The acknowledgement that we are in relationship with our bodies and minds is in itself a tool. Relationship involves polarity, each pole formed by the relationship with its opposite. Awareness of polarity is a fundamental tool of the mind. Polarity is a fact of life. It exists between and within cells. There is a polarity between self and non-self, inhalation and exhalation, tail bone and jaw, sacrum and occiput, male and female, you and I, and so on.

We work with the polarity, between tension and its release, gravity and the upward thrust from the ground,

the inner and outer body, centring and ex-centring, the left and right, voluntary and involuntary expression, doing and undoing, and between an experience and our awareness of the experience. We foster a dynamic balance between poles. If you are too much in your head you lose the sensitivity, if you are only in your body and lose the receptivity of the sensory mind, you have gone over the edge, you lose the thread.

There is no duality only polarity. Everything is unified by polarity. In the most cut off and encapsulated individual the polarity between self and universe is present but heavily weighted towards one pole. Thinking of one pole makes us aware of the opposite. Thinking of dark brings light to mind, thinking of love makes us aware of its absence. We are constantly reminded of the interplay between tension and its reduction. Opposites are always present when one or the other is in focus. Understanding polarity and how to work with it involves being aware of both ends of the spectrum simultaneously. This is the focus and the meditation.

Practice, like life, involves a polarity between direct and indirect action. Going into the body is direct action, receiving the consequence is indirect action. Direct and indirect action are inseparable poles of body-mind work. We may need to attend to one pole at any given moment but only to enhance the balance between both.

A fundamental polarity unites ancient qualities with current experience. The past is here, it is present. As we go into primal activity we awaken a past that moves into and through the present. A spontaneous spine and a fluid cord are presentations of an original state.

In the first few weeks the embryo is reaching outwards from a centre around which all activity revolves. Like a wheel around an axis. In the first week the embryo shows tendencies of consolidation with motion towards its centre. In the second week the opposite occurs, an opening towards the periphery. Centring is primary, expansion is secondary. Within the third week there is a gathering up of the inner body (Jaap van der Wal 2003).

The understanding that our most intimate relationship is with ourselves is the bedrock of all body-mind tools.

Impediments to Feeling Deeply

The quality of our responses relies on the quality of our sensations. The intelligence of an organism is determined by its sensitivity, which, in our case, may be impeded by our state of mind and physical condition.

'To be intelligent one must be aware of one's own impediments' (Krishnamurti 1954).

Krishnamurti's impediments refer to the mind and the factors impeding the quality of conscious awareness, attentiveness and sensitivity. These factors have just as much relevance with regard to the body. Many of us are unaware of our impediments until they lift. A lack of sensation is realised once the body has awakened.

Various factors conspire to inhibit sensitivity and the discovery of deeper movement. Basic physical tension reduces sensory awareness, but is not the only impediment. In our complexity, we unwittingly impede ourselves. Uninvited mental activity dulls sensitivity. The integral relationship between thought and feeling can be as counterproductive as it can be useful. Thought and its derivatives dull the sensory mind. Ambition, expectation, misplaced effort, anxiety and attachment to techniques are the products of non-essential thought. In the same way that we are the tool, we are also the impediment.

Methods and Techniques

Methods are reliable to a point but involve imitation. Someone initially *thought* of yoga. Its inception involved a mental construct focusing on deconstructing the habitual mind. At some point, the focus was also applied to the conditioned body. The body-mind work was, over time, fashioned into methods and techniques, an ongoing process that today produces a plethora of formulas. Methods have techniques, but both terms can mean the same. The Alexander Technique is a method and the Feldenkrais method is a technique. One can be methodical in one's technique and technical in one's method.

Habitual conditioning is easily exchanged for the conditioning of the method. You cannot surrender to primal action while engaged in a method unless you surrender the method. When something spontaneous occurs we may methodise it in order to own it, pass it on, or market it. This is normal, but there is no freedom in technique although technique may lead to freedom. Freedom lies in our ability to cooperate with an inherited behaviour and from releasing oneself to an inner intelligence. You are the authority on you. Only you know the quality and texture of your sensations.

A common distraction is a teacher's voice in your head, when they are no longer there or needed. The teachers do their job by providing a method that has been inspired by their teacher and/or comes from their own inspiration. Years after contact time with a teacher, he or she may still be there, in your head, in the practice with you. This is normal, particularly when something 'clicks': 'ah, that's what they meant'. This repetitive appearance may be confirmation that one is moving in the right direction, but then again, and with respect, perhaps it's time to move on. When one listens totally and exclusively to oneself there is no contradiction (or at least less of it). When we cling to another's teaching, we are not there; the natural self is pulled by an external energy.

We are our physical, psychological and emotional experience. We are in direct relationship with it. Only we can relate immediately to its continuous flow through direct communication with our own sensations, feelings, thoughts and evaluations. An original body presents itself to the individual that surrounds it, informing him or her of an intelligence common to the species, but that can only be experienced by personal inquiry.

As far as we can tell, there was/is no method to human development. The organism is more intelligent and more powerful than the methodology we use to reveal it. Mabel Todd writes: 'The imposition of a wilful "I" that attempts to force a change of behaviour upon the age old unconscious is futile. We only block habitual patterns of behaviour, which form the background of all present behaviour' (Todd 1953). In this context, Todd's 'habitual' refers to primal movement patterns.

We can only know what lies beyond methods by direct experience. A powerful intelligence lies beneath technique. It has no agenda, script or plan. It is inextinguishable from, but may be buried beneath, consciousness and need a little excavation. As it emerges it blows away all formulaic approaches. We need a structure to begin with, but the ideal technique dissolves technique.

Conditioning and Habit

Conditioning and habit encapsulate the original body by acting as an impediment to inner inquiry and outward expression. The traditional remit of yoga addresses conditioning and habit. Should we have the interest, this is the challenge. We have a resistance to change even when we invite it. The deeper our inquiry, the stronger is the challenge.

Conditioning and habit bury sensory wisdom, acting as a barrier to a deeper realisation. We are all conditioned by our past, and while some aspects may be positive other aspects have the potential for inhibiting physiological clarity. There is a fine dividing line between conditioning and habit. We are subject to conditioning but acquire habits. Some habit formation may be acquired as a consequence of our conditioning.

Conditioning may be reflected in a *cut off-ness*, while habit tends to disturb practice in the moment.

Conditioning, like tension, is essential. Tension is essential for physical survival and conditioning is essential for social survival. Certain patterns of tension and conditioning integrate because all conditioning necessitates patterns of tension that are laid down in response to the pressure of conformity. Conditioning itself implies a pattern of tension that is relative to the nature and extent of the conditioning. A fixed idea about life or a rigid adherence to a belief system has its own pattern of conditioning that is set in the pattern of tension related to it. It's a matter of degree; social, cultural, familial and educational conditioning are essential to a point but at what point might that point be beyond the best interests of the individual in terms of spontaneity, personal freedom and health.

Krishnamurti suggested that all memory, dormant or active, is conditioned. Habit and conditioning inhibit the movement of now. Our terms of reference exist in the past or the future. 'There are no *known* terms of reference in the now because there is nothing to refer to in the now' (1954). Sensation, however, is only in the now, although its quality may depend upon past events and circumstances.

The word *habit* comes from the Latin *habere*, meaning to hold. We all have habitual tendencies. We in-*habit* our bodies and may find preferential refuge in a shoulder, hip, or anywhere offering respite from unwanted feelings. Can you let go of your pelvis, suspend it freely from your spine for a sustained period? The habit of holding on to the pelvis may be so well-established that we cannot give it away, if at all, for more than a few moments without re-gripping it, because to do so involves giving up the habit of holding, just like that. We can't do it.

The fact that we are largely unaware of our conditioning is the essential feature of conditioning. It's not our fault, we have *been* conditioned. But we can detect habitual patterns in others and we may learn to sense them in ourselves. We might notice how they underpin ways of moving and being that lack ease and inner strength.

As practice is refined and the muscular aspects of conditioning begin to resolve, we may become more aware of the habitual behaviour that has been holding us back. Although habitual patterns may appear well ingrained they are external to the deeper possibilities. We can free ourselves, to some extent, by moving inwards beyond the encapsulation of past influence.

Identification and Ownership

Identity and the identification that comes with it are necessary but may also act as an impediment in practice. Identification may be empathetic, or self-referential. Self-referential identification is an impediment to the emergence of inner intelligence as it keeps the *me* in the foreground. Empathetic identification, on the other hand, fosters a more open attitude towards primal activity and its need for expression.

So much of what we do, we do to reinforce our identity. We could not function without names, labels, ownership or a direct sense of self. But accumulation props up our sense of self beyond that needed for security and invites an unwanted sense of separation. All our *prop*-erty, including others, ideas and practices, consolidates our sense of identity. We need an identity, but it can be exaggerated in and by practice preventing us from discovering deeper benefits.

My mat, belt, blanket, studio, of course, but in the same breath and with same sense of ownership, *my* yoga, *my* teacher, *my* students, philosophy, understanding, wisdom, exhalation, posture, spine, realisations, insights, hamstrings, *my* sensations, my-self. Of course, these *things* may be *mine* but only as a way in; the culture of *me* and *mine-ness* is an impediment to discovering a part of oneself that is free from identity and ownership. Perceiving one's body as one's property may be a reality but it's one that impedes practice, as it denies the existence of an intelligence that is not ours. We are the guests of this intelligence and have been given an opportunity to act accordingly.

The goal of meditation is to loosen the grip that identification has on the mind so that we are at least temporarily free from its insurgence. We can sense freely and openly into the body and receive its activity without the rust of identification.

Continual self-reference tends to reinforce the muscular patterns that give us the sense of ourselves. As important as it is to *be* ourselves, the quality of practice changes when we are immersed in a physical texture that leaves us behind.

Releasing the tension that holds us back involves dis-identifying with our sensations. Of course, we are guided by our sensations at all times, but when we perceive sensation as an intelligence in its own right the response is profound. When we free sensations from the grip of ourselves, when we de-possess them, they let us through and introduce us to an *entity* that is not caught up in id-*entity*.

Some people may be in therapy because they feel that they have no identity. They may need yoga or body work as a stabilising force, as an anchor from which to consolidate their sense of self before moving in a less attached direction. Primal movement is revealed by dropping the superficial me. We let go to an empowering force that arises from an unconditioned place. We discover an identity that is free from identification, at least for the time being.

Expectation and Ambition

It is only natural that the process contains some expectation and ambition during the initial stages of our inquiry and perhaps before each practice. If you begin sitting in meditation, you would *expect* any distractive ambition and expectation to evaporate. You would also *expect* to feel better as a consequence of the practice. If you are engaging in a deep physiological inquiry, going into your joints, soft tissues, breath, you have a goal, and you have expectation, otherwise you would not be there in the first place. The expectation based on past experience is that you will come back to a previously enlightening, refreshing, sometimes even extraordinary experience. The ambition is to deepen practice and make new discoveries, because you suspect or *know* they are there.

The depth body has no expectation or ambition other than to present its true, spontaneous and thought-less nature. Expectation and ambition are, within limits, natural elements that promote survival. The point is to be aware of the tendency, use it and drop it as primal activity emerges. Expectation and ambition may be unavoidable preliminary aspects of exploring your body, but are impediments when we are in the deeper work. The conditioning that restricts joints, shortens spines, traps energy and dulls experience is not just going to go away. Purposeful engagement with a healthy modicum of quiet expectation and ambition works well. But as our deliberations bear fruit, expectations and goal orientation dissipates as primal movement takes over.

When ambition meets the responsive nature of the organism the excessive tension reduces sensitivity and impedes progress. Physiology has no expectation, as it responds to the needs of the moment; its primary need is to be understood, and it can only be understood by listening to its requirements.

'To try and get it "right" by direct "doing" is to try and reproduce what is known, and cannot lead to the "right" as it is as yet unknown' (Alexander 1932).

Effort

Should we use effort, and if we use effort, what kind of effort should we use? Effort works well when it goes with the natural tendencies of the organism but works against us when it goes against these tendencies. It's easy to be too passive and just as easy to be overly tense. Passivity can lead to inertia, and excessive effort creates negative tension. We need to use physical effort in order to penetrate habitual tensional patterns, but should use it in the right way.

It is given that the mind is relaxed as it penetrates the working body but when should we work or relax the body? When we find the balance, we can experience the natural effort of primal movement emerge in response to the intelligent effort of our inquiry. 'The body works and the mind is calm' (Iyengar 1987).

The word 'effort' stems from the old French *esforcier*, 'force out'. The mechanical effort of trying to effect a position, which may restrict breathing and tighten the brain reinforces old patterns and blocks the ability to detect fine differences in the tissues. But there are times when an essential part of practice involves 'digging' into ourselves to bring out deeper activity. We need to sustain the action coming from the articulations; this takes work, and in this respect 'effort' is necessary.

Attention, vigilance, giving back to oneself, awakening sleepy or reluctant tissue and working with depth require necessary effort. But we are frequently unaware that we may be using too much effort. Misplaced effort pushes against the body instead of entering into it and acts as an impediment, inhibiting the natural effort needed by the deep body in the process of revealing itself.

Reactive or habitual effort (wrong effort) is based on an anxiety regarding what we want, on not being good enough, on competition, or on a conditioned inability to give up control. Unnecessary effort reinforces identity and expectation, increases resistance and impairs sensitivity. Right effort, as highlighted by the Buddhist tradition, focuses on refining positive qualities and eliminating negative ones. In this light, one can see attention as healthy effort, particularly if attention itself needs attention. Effort works well when it encourages the deep tension of unfolding from within and from the ground.

We are the authority on our tension levels and how to use our resistance. We can work and then relax and listen to the response of the tissues, followed by a period of more intensity, and so on. Any *practice*, by definition, requires attention. We can actively engage the diaphragm, draw the long bones towards the spine and then be more restful and let it happen. Attending to changes in tension and listening to the 'speech' of the body invite alternating effort with rest.

Non-essential Thought

It is obvious that thinking unrelated to the work at hand is superfluous and counterproductive. But when the body opens spontaneously, and moves from within, the thought that is related to the action at hand is also unhelpful, all thinking is superfluous. Even the mental registration of deep movement is counterproductive to the unreserved expression of the organism. 'When there is perfection there is no thinking; when there is no thinking, you are one with the truth' (Iyengar 1987).

We are thinking organisms but thought does not always have the organism's best interest at heart. Eastern *thought* perceives thought as heavy, as a concretion or thing. Thought inhibits the expression of the deeper body. We can feel this in ourselves; the more we think the more we become separated from the deep activity of the body, which existed long before the evolution of thought. As the body takes over, the experience is physiological. Deep action pushes thought to the periphery of our awareness. But thought is an opportunist and will reclaim its territory at the slightest chance. As sophisticated as the mind is, it cannot switch itself off, and in attempting to do so provokes more interference. We should be in control of thought, but it controls us; it is the tool that has taken over. It would seem intelligent to down tools when they are no longer needed.

When we are sensitive enough, we can feel thought as a tissue tension in the body. All thought is tension because thought is an activity requiring tension to act. Thoughts are also patterns of energy. James Oschman points out that the prefrontal cortex burns more energy than the basal ganglia or more ancient areas of the brain (Oschman 2000).

Thought provides a front door to a deeper experience, but can interfere once we are inside. As we work, we use thinking for reflection, introspection and evaluation but thought does not solve the problem of tension. Matthias Alexander writes: 'Knowledge concerned with sensory experience cannot be conveyed by the written or spoken word' (Alexander 1932). When we describe sensation to ourselves with thought words we prevent the finer activity from freeing itself for conscious awareness. Deep, fine and expansive behaviour is inhibited by thinking.

Sensation stimulates thought because we tend to recognise, describe and label sensation. If thought has evolved from an increasing awareness of sensory activity, it seems natural that sensory activity should stimulate thinking about the activity. Thinking arises when we describe sensations to ourselves with thought words. This is unavoidable because the thinking and sensory areas of the cortex are intimately associated. Sensory information registering in the neo-cortex is relayed to the rational cortex and translated into feeling — thought — words. My spine feels like this, my shoulder girdle that and so on. Analysis articulates the possibilities but is disruptive beyond a point. Thought has evolved out of its own activity. Thinking strengthens thought.

We can just let thought happen and pass on, and we do, but it is useful to be aware of the prevalent nature of thought while working into the body. During the rare

moments when thought is entirely absent, we become pure sensation. This experience enables the organism to expand beyond its habitual tendency.

Wilhelm Reich suggests that the organism has a biological need to express itself and that this need lies beneath recently acquired patterns of psycho-physical behaviour. He writes: 'The beginnings of living functioning lie much *deeper* than and *beyond* language. *Over and above this, the living organism has its own modes of expressing movement which simply cannot be comprehended with words*' (Reich 1933).

Thought defies simplicity because thought contains contradictory elements. Feeling is simple; you feel with an awareness that is uncluttered by activity. The cortex looks down into the body and the body looks up at the cortex. The body waits for a sign that the coast is clear; it waits for turbulence to abate so that it may reveal its hidden nature.

If the need arises, there are several ways of dealing with superfluous thought:

- Make friends with thinking and let it pass through you. *Fielding* incoming thoughts renders them outgoing as soon as they come in.

- When mental activity persists, return to thoughts connected to feeling. Describe the sensations to yourself as a way back in to thought-less-ness.

- When the power of the body surfaces, thought is blown away. This experience may be fleeting or more enduring. The body takes over the thinking mind as sensory realisation prevails.

We may think without language. Shadowy impressions, realisations and acknowledgements can exist without thought language, which is linear. Moshe Feldenkrais suggests:

Thinking is a much wider function which contains many forms of possible expression. Children can think before they can speak. We confuse speaking with thinking. Speech is a serial event, as words come one after the other in time and by their nature cannot communicate the thought which may contain an immense number of aspects. There is always more than one way of expressing a thought (Feldenkrais 2010).

Authentic, unconditioned experience is free from analysis and description, but might contain the shadowy presence of our distant observer, quietly in awe of the body's spontaneous activity. Thought cannot bridge the gap between itself and sensation. The art of *un-thinking* provides the sensory system with more space and energy with which to engage in its perceptions.

Krishnamurti observes: 'All thought is conditioned and thought cannot un-condition itself. But attention can. There is no method that can produce total attention. Total attention is not a result any more than love is. It cannot be induced or brought about by any action. An attentive mind is an empty mind' (Krishnamurti 1969). There is a point when all thought becomes superfluous, as an ancient language of the body presents itself to awareness.

Anxiety

Anxiety may pervade practice without our being aware of it. Low-grade anxiety is a feature of our culture. We may unwittingly take anxiety into practice and on occasion foster it. The feeling that things are 'not quite right' is endemic.

Practice takes the edge off of anxiety, or does it, and if so, to what extent? Yoga teachers are not exempt from seemingly unfounded anxiety, and they admit it. When asking a group who amongst them experiences anxiety on a regular basis, it is surprising how many raise their hands. It's not their fault and things might be worse had they not taken their chosen path. Yoga practitioners are no less vulnerable to anxious moments than anyone else. Life is not perfect; unease may be par for the course, what Krishnamurti and others might call a culture of fear. Ronnie Laing exclaimed: 'You can smell it [the fear] in the synovial fluid.'

The Eastern teachers suggest that unfounded anxiety (it is always founded) arises from knowledge which arises from thought. Once you follow the thinking path, you will at some point stir up a little anxiety about

something or other. Anxiety, like thought, is based on the past in relation to what we may expect from the future. I grew up in a family that always felt something bad was about to happen. Disaster could strike at any moment, and on the rare occasions that it did, they were proved right. So be prepared, be anxious in advance so that you are not taken by surprise. There is the anecdote about the Jewish woman who received an email from her mother, saying: 'Start worrying; details to follow.'

We can find anxiety anywhere in the body, in the knees, shoulders, jaw or in the breath. It acts as an impediment to deep expression. We may or may not be aware that low-grade unease/anxiety may surface in several ways as we practice:

- A low-grade habitual anxiety lying just beneath the surface that discharges as muscular patterns change.

- Anxiety arising from provoking tension — the body mind equates physical tension with a threat and reacts accordingly. Some people experience panic as their hamstrings grip them from behind.

- Anxiety that arises from 'losing oneself', i.e. letting go of the components that give us as a familiar sense of self such as, habitual tension, ideas and identification around the work. An unaccustomed sense of freedom can arouse a deep-seated fear of abandonment. Being in the void may provoke anxiety. The sense of emptiness and space when one is totally in the practice, when it is no longer a practice, may provoke feelings of anxiety related to 'not being there'. We may court freedom but can in reality be wary of it. There may be nobody at home! (In the true yoga tradition, there isn't.)

- An anxiety regarding getting it right, which stimulates negative effort and leads to working against the body, leading to more anxiety about getting it right.

- Deep-seated anxiety connected to past traumatic events may surface during or following practice. Body patterns acting as a safety valve release underlying anxiety into consciousness. Releases of this kind are supported by the practice, i.e. the contact with the ground and the strength of deep movement. Further change may manifest in dreams and ways of being.

- Current circumstances might carry an anxiety that is often alleviated in practice.

Plumbing our depths understandably stirs things up. Anxiety may be on a piece of elastic that lengthens as practice proceeds, but may spring back 'eventually'. The word *anxiety*, from the German root *angst*, taken literally means 'choking in the narrows'. We could posit that 'the narrows' might refer to the birth canal, and 'choking' the beginning of the uncertain and often stressful transition towards independent breathing. It could also refer to a constriction in the throat, trachea or the waist. These areas are often used to choke off unwanted feelings. When young, we can learn to control sexual impulses by pulling in the belly and fixing the diaphragm. Alexander Lowen writes: 'By constricting the waist we can cut off feelings of love in the heart from any direct connection to genital arousal' (Lowen 1958).

Cutting off feeling is not a selective process. Burying unwanted sensation suppresses desirable ones. Holding back fear, rage or frustration deadens feeling until feeling itself is inhibited. Someone having learnt how to hold back aggressive impulses will have also deadened the expression of love and the capacity to give and receive freely.

Freud noted the relationship between the obstruction to breathing and anxiety. This works both ways. Breath obstruction creates anxiety and anxiety creates breath obstruction. Apparently Freud did not follow up on his observations. Reich discovered the connection and did follow it up. Reichian work involving the breath is well known and documented (Reich 1933).

The practice of yoga can be equated (in a much milder way) with birth. The deep, transformational effect of yoga may arouse feelings that could be described as a rebirth. We come though ourselves from within as we unfold. A full uninhibited yoga or birth experience may be impeded by the onset of an anxiety that provokes negative muscular tension. Perhaps we are re-birthing ourselves, returning to a base state, an innocent way of being, free from conditioning, knowledge and its potential anxiety.

Anxiety is a feeling in the body that can be replaced by alternative feelings. We have an opportunity to take charge of anxiety patterns as they arise. Moving deeply inside the body might stir up feelings of anxiety but also enables us to confront them as we reinforce ourselves from a place within, free from anxiety and personal history. Our true centre is unconditioned, uncontaminated and untouched. Certain aspects of behaviour are founded on an anxiety. Time will tell whether or not the global interest in yoga is making a difference.

Time

The chronological perception of time works against us. Time is an impediment when we use it as a measurement or comparison, as something that occurs outside of us as opposed to being a part of us. Time impedes deeper inquiry when we use it as a division. The alternative experience of time implies no division; we are in flow, time ceases to be a *dur*-ation to be en-*dured*. (Both words stem from the Latin *durare*, meaning harden.) Being in time with time is to be in time with the organism which has no *idea* of time. We become aware of time as a movement, we are of time, in time and time is in us. Clock time has no feeling but *being time* can be sensed, and its ingredients include silence, calm and flow. When time no longer looks down upon us, we *are* time, free for unimpeded physiological expression. The body has no concept of time other than to move with it.

Jean Gebser, in his extraordinary book *The Ever Present Origin*, discusses Aristotle's view of time:

He [Aristotle] proceeds from the point of view that the 'Now' does not exist since it is at once the end of the past and the beginning of the future; consequently he considers it to be merely a kind of 'in between' which interrupts or interlinks as a fixed point in space and time without beginning or end (Gebser 1945).

Organic expression is hindered or facilitated by our relationship to time. Aristotle's observation supports the feeling of time as a movement. If *being* is a movement, time is the essential component of that movement. Our sense of being includes our sense of time, which is non-measureable. If we had no knowledge of time we would still have a flowing sense of it. Further to this and more relevant to practice is Aristotle's dismissal of 'the now'. We are given permission to let go of 'returning to the now' and can freely ride the movement of time.

Knowledge and Previous Experience

All knowledge, whether it be physiological, mechanical or philosophical, including what others have said, as useful as it may have been and perhaps still is, obstructs current sensory information. All past experience, however fruitful, is gone; we always start again and anew.

When we are not in the sensory mode, knowledge and past experience are necessary as they inform debate, invite analysis and support teaching skills. If we are in our own sensory mode while teaching, past experience and knowledge may come through on the back of current sensation. But in the intensity of deep movement, knowledge and reference to previous experience is unhelpful.

Reich writes: 'However, the living organism functions beyond all verbal ideas and concepts. Human speech, a biological form of expression at an advanced stage of development, is not a specific attribute of the living organism, which functions long before a language and verbal representation exist' (Reich 1942). Krishnamurti, a master of the 'unknown', continually suggests that what we know inhibits our possibility for growth.

Previous experience is connected to the past and arouses expectation and comparison. The stimulus for writing this certainly comes from knowledge and previous experience but when I am *in it* everything connected to the past is unhelpful, as it pulls me out of immediate experience. How long have we been practicing and teaching: 20, 40 years? All that experience up until the moments that are now passing. The weight of the past bearing down on the innocence of the organism, restraining an expression of movement that is free from previous workshops, teachers, certification, ideas and all that we know. In the process of going inwards we may encounter experiences that have, until then, been unknown. Referring to past experience buries the unknown beneath the weight of something that is gone, that is dead.

It is virtually impossible not to refer to something or another that is 'known' as we work through the layers of the body. The past and its accumulative knowledge provide the bedrock for further inquiry. Previous experience gives us a benchmark and a map from which to launch ourselves into something less known. The point is that we need to let go of it all as the more ancient intelligence arises. Knowledge and previous experience act as an initial key, but once used and the door is open, inhibit rather than enhance learning. The deep power of the body went about its business long before we knew about it.

Georg Feuerstein writes: 'Courage, then, is a matter of tapping into the core of our being — the Self — and allowing oneself to be dynamized and sustained by it'. The Swiss cultural philosopher Jean Gebser, referred to this attitude as "primal trust" or trust in the Origin, which is ever-present and inalienable (Feuerstein 1997).

Insensitive Pathways

Sensory flow moves centripetally, inward and upward towards consciousness. Sensory tissue is connected and supported by bone, fascia and muscle, and nourished by fluid. These elements interact to inform feeling, and an impairment of any one impacts upon the others, potentially reducing sensitivity.

Pathways to consciousness are affected by changes in the small spinal muscles, the diaphragm, thorax, limbs, extremities, and the general condition of the myofascial–skeletal system. Postural tension, habitual tension, scar tissue, personal history and health issues take their toll and influence sensory quality. Physical and psychoemotional factors combine to inhibit feeling. To reach awareness, sensory information travels through habitual tension plus the tension that may be provoked by the practice. Consider the distance that ankle sensation takes to reach consciousness and the potential resistance it may encounter on route.

The myofascial–skeletal system is rich in sensory receptors that record and register mechanical changes from moment to moment. The spinal cord receives sensory information, not all of which is relayed to the sensory area of the cortex. It is debatable what percentage of sensory activity might reach consciousness or what the potential for optimal input might be.

Deane Juhan, in his excellent book *Job's Body* writes: 'There is no one point along the afferent [centripetal] pathways or one particular level beneath the central nervous system below which activity cannot be a conscious sensation and above which it is a recognisable, definable sensory experience' (Juhan 1987). In other words, there is no clear demarcation between what can and cannot be felt. Sensitivity varies between individuals, particularly subtle activity, which is less amenable to the senses. The quality of feeling has the potential for considerable improvement. Frequent remarks are: 'I can't feel it', 'I can't make the connection', or 'That's amazing, I've never felt that before'. Our work clearly heightens sensation.

The nervous system provides a complex study and is still not fully understood. Countless sensory nerve endings are found deeply in connective tissue, joints and muscles. Traditionally, it is accepted that sensory impulses reach awareness via the spinal cord. Practitioners in the field of connective tissue reorganisation point to evidence suggesting there may be a faster sensory system at work, involving the transmission of information through the fascia. It is also suggested that fluid dynamics and its movement may contain liquid transmitters related to brain activity, giving another dimension to sensory receptivity.

Jaap van der Wal observes: 'The concept often prevails that joint receptors play the leading role in the process of monitoring joint position and movement for the purpose of statesthesis and kinethesis while muscle receptors are regulated to motor functions that operate at a subconscious or reflex level' (van der Wal 2012).

This observation is supported by Deane Juhan, who writes:

Our muscles, seventy to eighty-five percent of our physical bulk, deliver to us very little sensation that we can consciously identify, and if we block with a local anaesthetic the sensations arising from the skin and the associated joint capsules, we have no feeling whatever for where our limbs are in space, or what sort of movement they are up to (Juhan 1987).

If this is correct, we feel our bodies through the agency of nervous tissue associated with fascial tissues, particularly those in and around joints. It does feel that muscle gives us a direct sense of stretch, contraction and release, but then muscle is heavily invested in fascia.

The conveyance of sensory information may vary in form but we can still assume that nervous activity is paramount, that it moves towards the brain, and is prone to interference. Symptoms of spinal nerve entrapment include paraesthesia, numbness or pain. Recent research may shed light on mechanisms that speed up sensory conduction, but pressure on a spinal nerve may seriously modify sensation within the area of its distribution.

We can feel the consequence of sensory activity but not the actual conduction. Our perception of weight, pressure, tension, contraction, space, rhythm, release and the relationship of body parts in space, to each other and to the ground, are processed beneath awareness.

Tissue sensation moves towards and through the spinal cord, lower and mid-brain and registers in the upper centres of consciousness. Informed responses travel from the centre back to the tissues. Sensation and responsive action are inseparable. Nervous action responding to incoming sensory information provides further sensation which in turn modifies and influences subsequent responses. At the most basic level, an endless flow of sensation and action gives us our muscle tone, general body sense and sense of self.

The nervous activity supporting the body against gravity is largely inherited and occurs beneath conscious awareness. The nervous system is not fully wired at birth and is also influenced by one's environment. Nervous activity instilled by learning and the formation of habit is acquired through and beyond infancy. Acquired behaviour sinks beneath a conscious level as more complex operations take precedence. This forms the bedrock of conditioning and, depending on the circumstances of early life, can inhibit feeling.* We are unaware of the 'dulling down' process and may not understand why sensations available to others elude us. The point is that incoming sensation having the potential to be 'felt' might be conditioned, and give us limited sensory readings. (The writing of Moshe Feldenkrais makes essential reading in this respect.)

*Most of us are familiar with a childhood sensation of 'butterflies' in the belly, which is an unsuccessful attempt to suppress unwanted feelings.

Nervous transmission has been compared to electricity, but transmission also has a chemical element that assists conduction across interconnecting nerves. Hormonal input from the body-mind such as adrenaline, which suppresses sensitivity, and endorphins, which enhance it, also play a part in the physiology of feeling. Adrenaline-charged practice inhibits feeling.

Physiologists describe three main phases of sensory activity: 1) local sensation; 2) integration, selection and modification within the nervous centres, the highest being the brain and the highest in the brain being the sensory/motor cortex; and 3) the release and direction of coordinated impulses to effect the appropriate motor response of the body.

The area between the sensory and motor areas of the cortex (middle association area) is said to make up approximately 90 per cent of the entire nervous system. This area influences the responsive outcome of sensory input and is said to be responsible for the evolution of consciousness. This information supports the experience that heightened physiological sensitivity contributes to an enhanced quality of consciousness. As the body awakens, we awaken with it. The sensory association area of the cortex also stores memory of past sensory experience enabling us to compare current sensations with previous experience.

Physiologists also identify a *secondary sensory pathway* descending *from the cortex* that can inhibit or facilitate incoming sensations. This pathway gives sensitivity to the incoming sensory pathway as the information comes in and is influenced by *past experience* and the nature of the stimulation at the time. It also enables us to give our attention to single sensations in the presence of many other sensations and allows us to choose a sensation to focus on. The sensitivity of this pathway and the efficiency of its transmission are influenced by our general state, our personal history and what is happening at the moment of transmission. This important component of our sensory mechanism gives different people varying experience of the same stimulus and may even choose to highlight or block out a potential sensation (Tortora & Anagnostakos 1990).

In other words, a descending sensory pathway emanating from the conscious brain accepts or rejects incoming sensations. The outcome depends on 'how we are' at the time, and on previous experience and personal history.

A primary somesthetic (soma = body, aesthesis = perception) or general sensory area of the cortex also has a relevant function in relation to what sensations we perceive and how we can perceive them. The size of each sensory area of the brain receiving information from the various parts of the body is related to the number of receptors in that part of the body, not the size of the part; for example, the sensory area receiving information from the lips is large compared to a relatively small sensory area receiving information from the thorax. We might use the lips in practice; softening them has the effect of softening the entire system, perhaps because their large number of sensory receptors influences the sensory climate of the body as a whole. The thorax, on

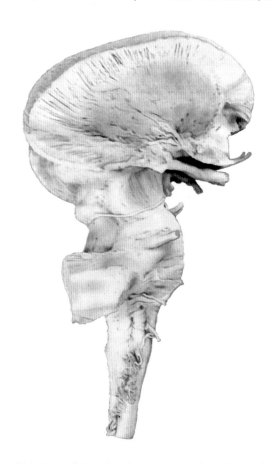

Figure 8.1

Sensory input – brain stem as a creature.

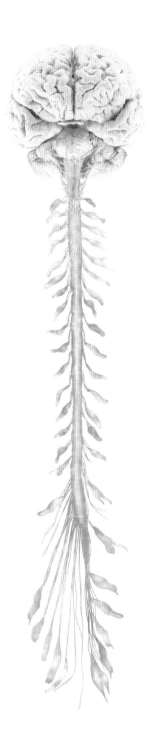

Figure 8.2

Spinal nerves, cord and brain as a creature.

the other hand, is a primary focus in practice but has relatively fewer sensory nerve endings. Perhaps we should combine a sensory awareness of the lips and thorax in practice: one nervous system, one sensory spread.

The locations of the common integration area or gnostic area (gnosis = knowledge) are closely linked with somesthetic association areas. The gnostic area receives impulses from the somesthetic area and integrates sensory interpretations from the association areas and impulses from other areas so that a common thought can be formed from various sensory inputs. It then transmits signals to other parts of the brain to cause the appropriate response to the sensory signal. This basic link sheds light on the relationship between sensing and thinking. Our thinking inhibits sensation. Sensory awakening dissolves thought.

The association areas of the cerebrum and cortex connect sensory and motor areas and are also connected to memory, reasoning, will, personality traits, intelligence and emotions. *Knowing* this supports the realisation that how we are, in our practice, influences the quality and depth of what we are feeling. Experience shows that sensory input is inhibited when the cortex is overloaded, busy or simply dull.

Excessive or chronic muscular tension is incompatible with feeling clearly and deeply. Tissue loses sensitivity through overload. Postural factors and past physical trauma may inhibit sensory awareness. Nervous tissue is vulnerable to strain, mechanical stress, compression and distension and is susceptible to pressure from neighbouring and surrounding structures such as bone, muscle, tendon, ligament or fascia. Nerves, when subjected to excessive mechanical stress, might respond by becoming overstimulated, but, when the stress is prolonged, become fatigued and underactive, leading to a reduction in sensitivity.

We do not *feel* the underlying activity of the sensory system and cannot distinguish the areas concerned as they go about their sensory business. But we are more than aware that sensation flows into consciousness. The above information is supportive. Our work addresses sensitivity, and its scope is wide open. Practitioners of long standing, in their 80s and 90s, awaken subtleties of action and sensation that were previously dormant. The essential factor in 'feeling more' is being totally attentive to what you can feel, and letting the sensations in with as little mental interference as possible. We may have impediments to deep sensation, but can use them as doors to a deeper experience.

Taking into account all that is said and known regarding sensory activity, we can view the nervous system as an organ within an organism. Taking the brain, brain stem and the spinal nerves out of situ they appear as creatures in their own right. This is reflected in their natural design. (Figures 8.1 and 8.2) If we did not know that they represented the human nervous system we can appreciate them as a primal intelligence, with or without the organism that surrounds them.

Doors

Doors to Expression

If we were free from impediments there would be no yoga; there would be no need to practice anything.

Impediments are our best teachers; they give us doors to pass through and invite a transcendental process. A door is an appropriate metaphor, as we can pass through and beyond a threshold. The door does not close behind us but remains open, enabling us to pass either way.

We may classify impediments (or not) as we work. In general terms *we are the impediment*. By directly approaching impediments, by being fully aware of them and entering into the *feeling* of them, they dissipate. We can pass through ambition because we experience it. But we cannot directly enter the source, the neo-cortex, because we don't feel it. We might visualise the structure of the cortex and its functions but this changes nothing because the cortex is not an experience. We experience the con-sequence of neocortical activity but not the cortex itself. We address the neocortex by addressing its conditioned responses. The cortex is unaware of its own conditioning but we are aware of our condition-ing through the agency of the cortex.

Going into and through an impediment enables an entry to a deeper activity. We can go through each and every door as it appears. Doors re-present themselves like Russian dolls, each time at a deeper level, until we find ourselves free from obstructions. Everything taking up residence in the body/mind is external to the deep activity it surrounds.

'Passing through' is the common experience. We may pass through tension, sluggishness, weakness and turbu-lence. We can pass through psychological doors at will, but how deep are the physiological doors? We can move into and pass through the spine time and again. A physi-ological door is a sensation; we pass through what is felt.

You can pass through impediments, and then pass through the acknowledgement of passing through them because each acknowledgement is the next impediment; in other words, we are never free from ourselves unless we stop experiencing. Frank McLynn, in his biography of Jung writes:

He [Jung] said that it was impossible to gain the state of being 'not-conscious' while alive and still be able to remember it, as Hindus claimed. Patiently he argued that you could not get rid of the idea of ego even in the deepest state of samahdi, for the moments of existence would have been non-existent and left no memory trace (McLynn 1996).

In terms of *our* inquiry, it may be sufficient to dissolve our conditioning, wipe the slate clean momentarily and swing between the poles of conscious appreciation and organic innocence.

Going in is the precursor to coming out and is the first stage of unfolding. Impediments to going in also impede the possibility of coming out. A closed door inhibits movement in both directions; an open door provides a two-way possibility. *The mind penetrates imped-iments on the way in and the depth body penetrates them on the way out, giving the feeling of tissue and consciousness unfolding in one movement.*

Passing Through

We have choices:

- Ignore rogue activity and let it take care of itself. This may fill you up, as activity combines with action, leaving little space for reflection.

- Field the activity (of the mind), deflect it and continue to explore. The acknowledgement of exploration can also obstruct progress (I am now exploring etc.).

- Impose a practice on the activity, e.g. the breath, sound, an idea. These are distractions that might create an impasse.

- Surrender all thoughts, ideas, concepts, realisations, physical tensions, weight; surrender the idea of surrendering and start again.

- We can celebrate our impediments and lighten up. Celebration works — when we *go in*, we are celebrating life, but premature celebration does not change well-established patterns. The organism responds to an unreserved respect that may involve some seriousness. To work inside your self is an undertaking. We have not accumulated our impediments lightly; in one way or another we pay a price for carrying them. We do the work, open up, and celebrate as celebration arises by itself, but not by pretending.

- We can acknowledge the nature of impeding factors as they arise, and go directly into and through them. Cutting through an impeding factor with the laser of the mind, being attentive to it, may be a reminder that its foundations are not as strong as first thought. Directly cutting through impeding factors renders them redundant immediately and enables a more primal activity to cut through impeding factors from inside out.

On the physical level, we can go into the body through entry points. The skin is easily accessible. Freud proposed that the development of the ego-self begins as a direct result of sensations on the surface of the body. Releasing and working with the skin alters one's sense of self, and takes us to a deeper place. Skin sensations can be directed inwards towards the spine. We can enter the body through contact points with the ground: elbows, forearms, shoulders, wrists, ribs, heels, pelvis, sacrum, dorsal spine, or anywhere acting as a gravitational base.

Have no previous experience, be a guest of time. Time has no problem with itself because it is in time with itself. Remain receptive, as the sensations come towards you, do not *know* them. Give up a sense of owning the practice. Pass through personal relationship to what you feel.

Two voices of authority pass through you, the voice of others and what they have said, and your own voice, the authority of your own experience. When the voice of others dissolves you are left with your own voice; when your own voice dissolves you are in an original experience.

Thinking cannot let go of itself; there is not one thing that you can think about that can release you from thinking. But going into thought with pure perception dissolves thought and sends it to the periphery of your awareness. Losing your mind enables your sensory mind to take over. The 'brakes' of cortical control are taken off as subcortical expression reveals itself. The natural behaviour of your spine may expunge thinking, but you must catch it. At some point, pure awareness takes over, an awareness devoid of thinking.

As involuntary movement arises, ideas about postures and the inner verbalisation accompanying them drop away. Deep movement spreads throughout one's total being. Moving in time with time releases the creative impulse; creative practice is being the practice. We may try this angle, or make that adjustment, but unconditioned creativity occurs within the uncontainable flow of time. The movement of the mind with the body is totally creative when it is free from conditioning because the flow of the past into the future through the body-mind is creative. We are in creation.

Noticing how we are in ourselves and in relationship involves modifying impulses and censoring thoughts and feelings. This kind of transcendence, instilled by socialisation, is not so different from transcendence in practice. The propensity to *go beyond is in us*. Jean Gebser refers to the observation of George Simmel, who wrote: 'transcendence is imminent in life' (Simmel 1945).

There is a point, just before, just as, the organism opens up, when the tendency to interfere is particularly prevalent. This tendency occurs as the body-mind invites us to pass through itself — here comes — there goes — stiffness — other people — ambition — resolution — success — self-satisfaction — here comes — there goes — stiffness — other people — ambition — we accept the invitation.

Breathing: The Ultimate Tool

The Ultimate Tool

The breath is the deep inquirer, a practitioner in its own right. Sensitive or powerful, quiet or voluminous, the breath awakens the depth body and leads us towards an unknown experience.

The breath is second only to feeling as an instrument for going inward and for stimulating original movement. Breathing feels its way into articulations, activates tissue, moves fluid, and finds its way in to our deepest recesses.

Breathing and movement on land developed simultaneously. As we crawled, crouched and stood, we breathed. Our primal ancestors breathed into their depth bodies millions of years before the advent of thought and the implementation of biomechanical laws. We breathed with a primitive thorax and diaphragm before the development of limbs. Breathing and its depth were instrumental in our progression from all fours to standing. The evolution of breathing and its current practice can both be seen as processes of refinement.

The baby in utero produces the thoracic movements of breathing, a natural practice for post-natal life. Jaap van der Wal writes:

Bodily functions, physiological functions, psychological functions are pre-exercised as growth gestures and growing movements in the embryo. In this respect a human being has already breathed long before he has taken his first breath after birth. The dynamics – in the sense of the gesture of morphological development

– with which lungs, thorax, and diaphragm are developing and unfolding, may be considered and interpreted as a type of breathing because they are breathing movements. The breathing of an embryo is not yet breathing air in a physiologic way, but it represents a more fundamental breathing in a morphological way, in form so to speak (van der Wal 2003).

Breathing is intimately tied to deep skeletal movement. The breath moves the spine and the spine moves the breath. A visitor to Martha Graham one evening found her experimenting on the floor. He left, and on returning the next morning found her in similar mode. She had been finding out how much her body would move by only using her breath.

The breath is mechanically and rhythmically connected to the entire body through connective tissue, soft tissue, bone and fluid. Breathing touches and activates spinal articulations, the girdles and the limbs. Deeper breathing creates deeper feeling because it creates movement from within, and movement enables feeling. A deep breath is not a matter of volume of air inspired. A deep breath touches and moves the spinal discs and facet joints, the small intersegmental muscles, and moves out into the long bones and extremities. The breath and the spine move each other.

Impediments to an Original Breath

The breath is impeded by the same factors that obstruct access to the deep body, as seen in Chapter 8. High on this list is our use of respiratory muscles to 'hold ourselves together'. The location, nature and strength of the diaphragm and abdominal muscles are perfectly suited for holding down feeling. Feeling is suppressed by consciously or unconsciously adjusting our breath. Breathing patterns may be established by personal history or birth experience. The quality of our first breaths may instil respiratory patterns that can continue into adulthood.

There may be as many imbalances and tensions in the breathing mechanism as in the musculoskeletal system as a whole. A weak or stiff diaphragm may restrict the end of exhalation and limit the next intake of breath (I can't get inspired). Some people may be held at the end of inhalation (I can't let go). Both tendencies inhibit the diaphragm's ability to work deeply with the spine and the body as a whole. Practitioners discover that they hold on somewhere within their breathing cycle and that working to free the breath also activates deep movement.

Physical restrictions limit the potential depth of the breathing. Respiratory freedom is inhibited by fixations or stiffness between the thorax, spine and ribs, or a lack of elasticity in the costal cartilages or around the shoulder and pelvic girdles. Discrepancies in the lumbar spine, sacroiliac joints and hips may restrict the work of the diaphragm. The entire spine functions as a respiratory organ and stiffness between vertebrae restricts deep expansive breathing potential. The thoracic spine represents the back of the thorax and is particularly relevant to respiration. Even restrictions in the feet and hands can have implications for the chest cage and respiratory muscles. Figure 10.3C is a reminder of respiratory hands and feet actively receiving from and giving to the central respiratory mechanism (See page 75).

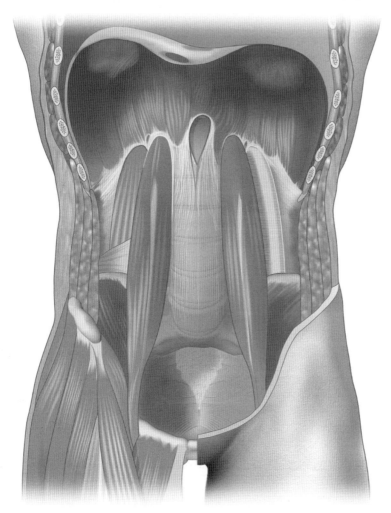

Figure 10.1

The central mechanism.

We might be unaware of the extent of restrictions in elasticity and breathing space until they are resolved, and might be surprised at the profound relationship between breathing and primal movement once the restrictions have lifted. Working with the breath and other elements of postural practice dissolves many inhibitive fixations. Mabel Todd writes: 'In primary patterns of movement, in the absence of structural fixities superimposed by man, the breathing apparatus and the locomotive apparatus interrelate, aiding one another. This must be so since locomotion and breathing developed movement and form together' (Todd 1937).

Five Choreographies

When directing, and being directed by, breathing movements we are presented with at least five distinct yet overlapping choreographies:

1. Voluntary organisation of bones; for example, arranging and rearranging your arms to release the upper spine and open your rib cage. Changing contact points with the ground will enhance breathing by releasing tension where and when needed. The possibilities are numerous and the benefits best accrued by creative inquiry.

2. Harnessing involuntary internal breathing movements. The nature of each breath is unpredictable and invites us to work with its inherent intelligence.

3. An outwardly expressive involuntary movement occurs when the spine and breath coordinate. This action transmits into the arms and legs, and the entire body moves spontaneously. These movements vary in intensity and direction.

4. The spine flexes on exhalation and extends for inhalation. In the all-fours position the tail and head move towards and away from each other. This literally looks as if we are coming up for air as the head lifts for the in breath. Reich comments on this: 'As soon as the diaphragm expands and contracts freely, i.e. respiration functions fully and spontaneously, the trunk strives with each exhalation, to fold up in the region of the upper abdomen. In other words: the neck end strives forward towards the pelvic end' (Reich 1942). Reich considers this movement in relation to his interest in the 'orgasm reflex' but in our terms this is a primal movement and relevant to our return to a freer physiological state. Respiratory flexion and extension of the entire spine can be found in all positional work.

5. We can 'pump' the breath at a faster pace to move the spine into more dynamic waves. This practice involves actively lifting the diaphragm on exhalation. The abdominal muscles follow the action and are sucked back towards the spine and then released completely for the inhalation. This practice should only be used in short bursts followed by slow and spontaneous breathing, in order to feel the subsequent changes in space and depth.

This work is exploratory and creative and defies methodisation due to the unpredictable nature of the organism. The requirements change as moment-to-moment feeling changes.

The Exhalation and Going Inwards

The outbreath is experienced as a centripetal movement as the expulsion of air draws all tissues towards the spine. The thorax, diaphragm and internal rib tissue cohere to take you inwards. The diaphragm is a deep and powerful coupling between the thoracic and abdominal cavities and is the essential agent in exhalation. Its deep, strong lumbar fibres (the crura) have an important influence on the spine.

Muscles and connective tissue work as a unit *led by the diaphragm*. When unimpeded, the diaphragm creates an *upward and inward draw* on the out-breath. The tissue lining the inside of the thorax is felt significantly and we should be aware that the belly always *follows* the diaphragm on exhalation. It is not necessary to list the action of all the muscles involved in breathing. The body functions as a whole and its respiratory activity is no exception. The main features of exhalation are that the diaphragm sucks up and back, followed by the deep muscles of the waist and the belly as a unit. You can feel the components of the central mechanism acting as *one powerful rhythmic organ*. Figure 10.1 gives a visual sense of the deeper aspects of the central mechanism in relation to respiration and deep body control.

'The diaphragm is the most important anterior muscle of the spine, but do not tell Westerners this or they will use it like a muscle' (Iyengar 1987). Although this good advice from Iyengar holds true, we need to work for diaphragmatic efficiency. The diaphragm can be weak and stiff and might take a little application before it can spread its wings naturally. Figure 10.4 gives a strong visual sense of the presence of the thoracic diaphragm. It looks as it might feel, a powerful central organ with extraordinary versatility and the potential for moving the entire body.

Deep respiratory action engages and opens articulations, moves bones and activates soft tissues. We can foster this action to good effect in all positions and movements. During the transition from exhalation to inhalation, the gathering of all tissue connecting to the diaphragm gives deep control to the central mechanism as it unfolds for inhalation. The power of this action opens out through the spine, into thorax, shoulders, arms, hands, pelvis, legs and feet. The dynamic interweave between articular movement, myofascial integration and breathing is one complete ancient movement.

Working the Breath

We can breathe in any position but those in Figure 10.3 are well suited for releasing the anti-gravity muscles, giving them more freedom to engage with the breath.

To maximise the potential of the exhalation for supporting deep postural control and movement it is necessary to release negative tension and engage positive tension while working in to the deeper action of the breath that comes from the front of the spine.

The pelvic and shoulder girdles should release by dropping weight through their contact points. The diaphragm has no direct contact points with the ground but is stimulated by bones that do. Spinal, rib, shoulder and pelvic points are all effective. Abandon your weight to the ground, your exhalations to the spine, and your mind to the sensations. This is where the juice is.

Remember to make a soft hissing noise around your epiglottis. This creates a valve-like action in your throat, giving your diaphragm, abdominal and pelvic floor muscles a little resistance to work against, promoting their effect locally and throughout the body. Pursing the lips in a whistling attitude can be an alternative.

Activate the mechanism with purposeful breaths and then allow the natural action to take over. When depth becomes shallow and weakens, you can reintroduce purposeful breaths. An expansive breath may be followed by several smaller ones which are just as deep, sometimes even more so, because the system is open and receptive. When the exhale disappears inside you, allow it to return in its own time and its own way. The spine draws the breath and the breath moves the spine.

Breath-guiding Awareness

- Use the breath to feel the relationship between your bones, articulations and tissues. Feel the shape and versatility of your thorax, pelvis and spine. Feel through the front of your thoracic and upper lumbar vertebrae and the fluid response of your entire spine and sacrum. Follow the action wherever it takes you. Encourage the gathering sensations inside the rib cage, and out into the shoulders. The action of your belly following your diaphragm spreads out into your superficial connective tissue and skin.

- Don't breath in until it arrives from deeply inside you; wait for depth to take over and move from inside out.

- Follow your exhalation into your spinal discs and the small intervertebral muscles; they are present and active! Keep your jaw relaxed, and slightly open, to receive the action coming up through the cervical spine.

- Centre the femoral heads in their sockets to connect with the shoulders. Give your arms and legs back to the spine, enabling it to move from a deeper place, creating more space within the thorax.

- The soles of the feet and palms of the hands work as accessory diaphragms. Feel their tension come and go as the fingers and toes pick up the impulse to work. Activate your big toes, which are directly connected to your pelvic floor and diaphragm.

- Wait for incoming breaths to arrive from the roots of the diaphragm and deep lumbar spine. As you empty on exhalation, move your awareness into the space arising from your deep waist, pelvis and chest.

General Respiratory Sensations

- There is a general feeling of expansion before inhalation. The core of the body opens out in all directions towards the surface. Mechanically, it is all one movement. The tail and pubis approximate, the thigh bones and upper arms rotate externally, the lower tips of the shoulder blades rotate towards each other and the thoracic spine moves inwards.

- Return to the feeling of integration and inner space. Follow the shape of the skeleton and feel the breath play through the large pelvic, abdominal and thoracic spaces.

- Remain grounded on the inhalation. This is a major challenge in practice, as our conditioning will continually try to reassert itself. As you exhale, consolidate your contact points and draw towards your centre.

- Purposefully or quietly, breathe your breath and feel it inside you. Watch it change its rate and rhythm. Give your breath to your body and your body to your breath.

- Finally, give more attention to the location and shape of your tail — it comes to life — flexing and extending

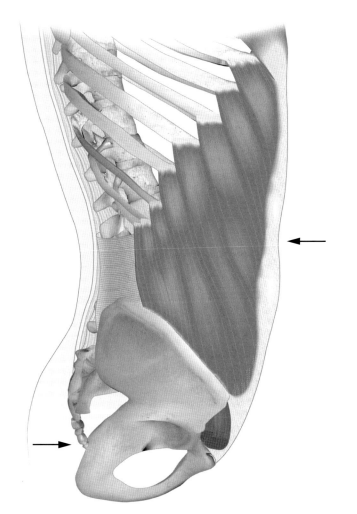

Figure 10.2

Abdominal tissue – tailbone and breathing.

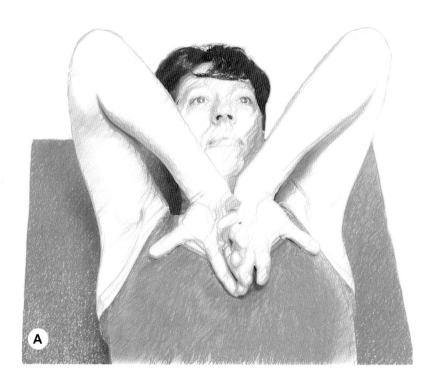

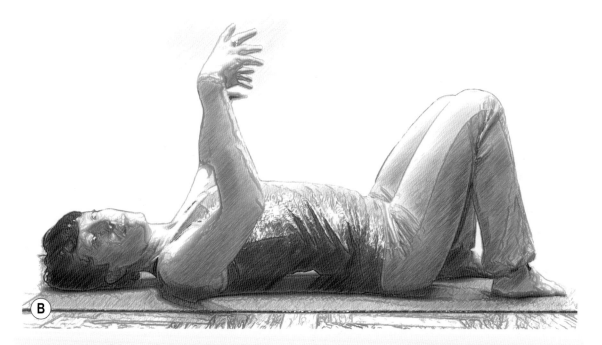

Figure 10.3 A and B

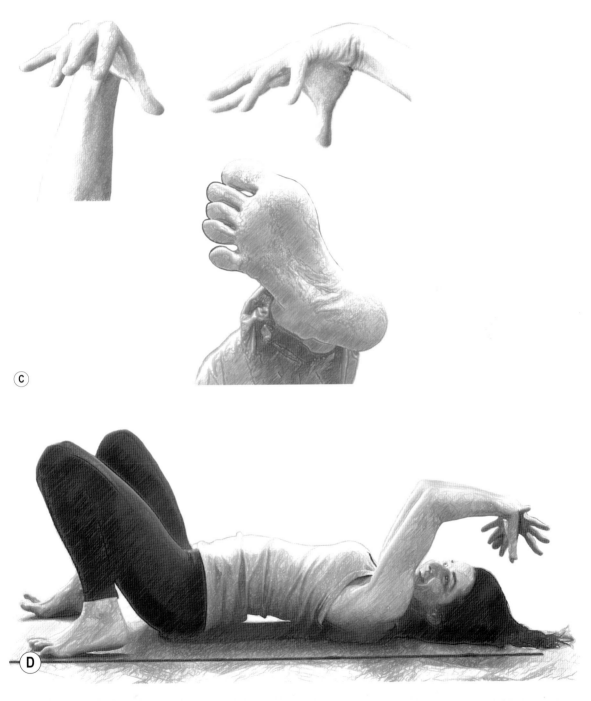

Figure 10.3 C and D

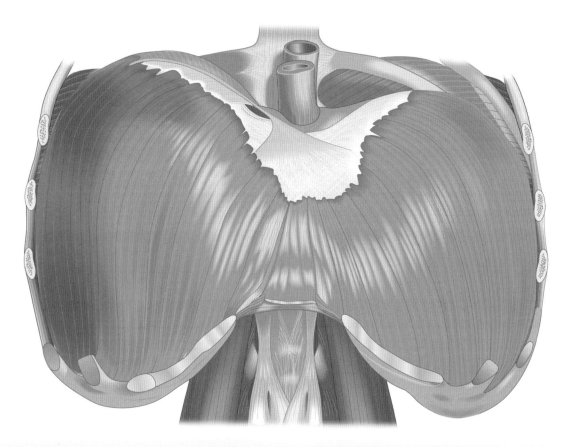

Figure 10.4

The diaphragm as an organ.

rhythmically — fluidising the sacroiliac joints and all the vertebrae above — the tail bone holds the key to the relationship between respiratory and spinal mechanics. The tail and pelvic floor act as a pump that stimulates the whole system. Figure 10.2 reminds us of the working relationship between the abdominal muscles and the tail bone. We can acknowledge and encourage this relationship in all positions.

Mechanical and Chemical Intelligence

We cannot possibly know when we need the next in breath unless we are reading a device that registers our blood chemistry. The chemical needs of the blood and the mechanics of deep movement have evolved simultaneously and should continue to cooperate. Mabel Todd writes:

The breathing apparatus and the timing mechanism relating breathing rhythms to skeletal rhythms are developed to meet the need for getting oxygen to all the deep body cells, burning up in the activities of living and this is done with complete harmony between the rhythms of the two systems (Todd 1937).

When carbon dioxide levels reach a certain level, receptors in the brain stem and lungs provoke a reflex that *inspires* inhalation. We cannot feel the activity of these receptors but we can feel the consequence of their intelligence. We can feel the deep transition from exhalation to inhalation, and the sensitivity needed to allow this process to take place without interference.

If we do not give this process enough time for chemical exchange at the level of the lung tissue, we tend to block the clear exchange of gases and restrict the depth of breathing needed to open the spine and thorax. The stimulus for opening occurs in advance of the incoming breath as the mechanism opens for inhalation. The body is not expanded *by* the in breath but expands *for* it.

Deeper Still

Breathing is not only a tool for body work but is also a practice in itself, although it can be seen exclusively as body-work because of its effect. An *original breath* is free from the constraints of personal patterns, has no agenda other than to express itself and is not tethered by ideas of what it should or should not do. No two breaths are the same in quality, texture, depth or impact. Breathing intelligently recognises the process *as* an intelligence. Wilhelm Reich's reference to the intelligence of the organism can be applied to the breath:

It is simply impossible to translate the language of the living organism directly into the word language of consciousness. It is extremely important to realize this, for the rationalistic thinking which has shaped man's mechanistic civilisation is capable of smothering and extinguishing our insight into the fundamentally different language of the living organism (Reich 1942).

Slipping out of knowledge is essential in rebalancing the tensional quality of your breath. An original breath is not bound by constructs but arises through quiet and penetrating attention. The pause is not passive but is a profound organic movement, which on occasion may seem endless (is an inhalation ever going to arrive?).

Allow the exhalation to slip into your spine. Small rhythmic, movements may occur during the longer pauses as the mechanism resets itself. Within these small movements you may notice micromovement and fluctuating nuances, indicating a delicate intelligence at a deeper level.

The tail, sacrum and sacroiliac joints breathe, soften and pulsate and we can feel their influence through the spine and ultimately the whole body. As the exhalation draws the body towards the centre and we wait, the inhalation arises from within the spine; it comes by itself. The natural tension between the out- and in-breath is an expression of unfoldment.

The deep respiratory mechanism is never silent, a continuum without end or beginning. The art of non-interference is put to the test before the inhalation arrives. The combined effect of attention, undisturbed composure and organic intelligence enables us to move from a new place and in a different way.

A Respiratory Dance

You can invite your bones to dance by using an exaggerated approach that frees the body in a remarkable way. *Releasing for the in-breath and gathering with the out-breath in a more demonstrative way stimulates an articular dance.* A spontaneous choreography performs myriad activities. The breath and spine dance together, and every vertebra dances with its neighbours. The shoulder blades dance with the collarbones and spine; the long bones dance with their girdles. The thorax, diaphragm and spine become one undulating organ as their texture melds into softness and fluidity.

Place your hands face up on your breast bone (Figure 10.3A). At first, breathe deeply and purposefully, and then allow it to happen. The thoracic spine moves forward, following the lumbar spine in extension as the spine prepares for the in-breath. Eventually, your hands will separate and your arms unfold *by themselves*, as your shoulder blades move in and the collarbones separate in response to the forward and inward movement of the spine. As you proceed, you notice that there is no division between moving bones and breathing. You move into something beyond cortical direction, an ancient expression of life that we can only wonder at.

Not Knowing the Breath

Not knowing, owning, or anticipating the breath invites extraordinary freedom and inner space. When the out-breath enters this space and *has completely left you*, you immerse into a primal and innocent place. The breath has moved you into an alternative intelligence, and you find yourself suspended in the unknown. The twentieth-century German philosopher Husserl suggested that: 'The essence of a thing resides not in its actuality but in its possibilities' (Husserl 1949). This insight reflects a spatial depth that contains the *possibility* of an inhalation.

An organic breath is an event. It is the personal experience of an impersonal occurrence. We pass through concepts about breathing and meet an unconditioned, depersonalised and original breath coming towards us. Respiratory mechanics fall away as rhythm, fluidity and a profound sense of inner unity and connection to the external environment take over. The breath has the potential for bringing into play what Reich called the 'sensation of totality'. Totality not only refers to the integration of physical feeling, but also to the integration of body, mind, emotion and environment. The sensation of totality moves us beyond the confines of ourselves and is a primal experience.

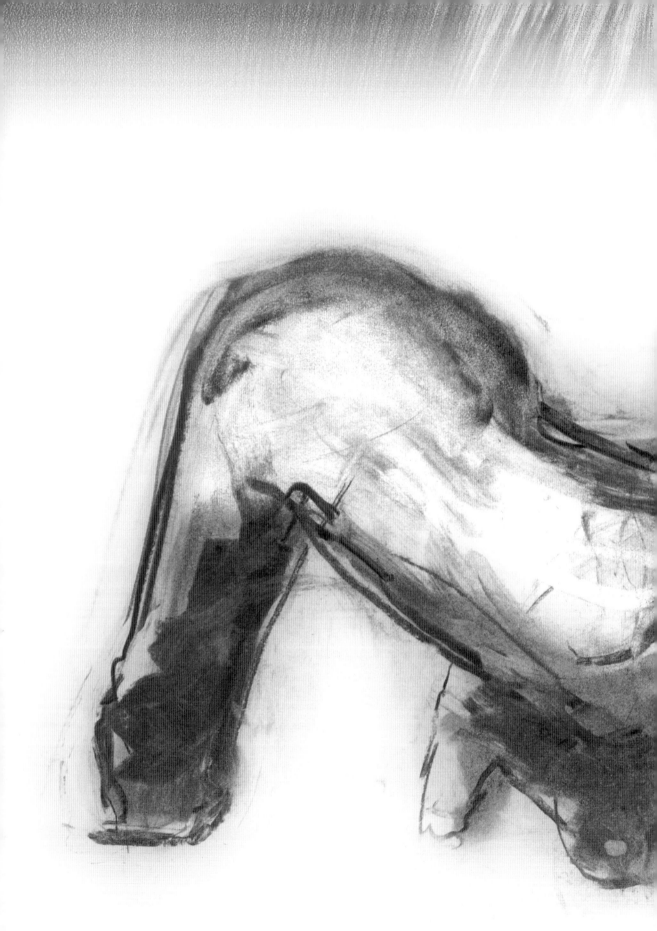

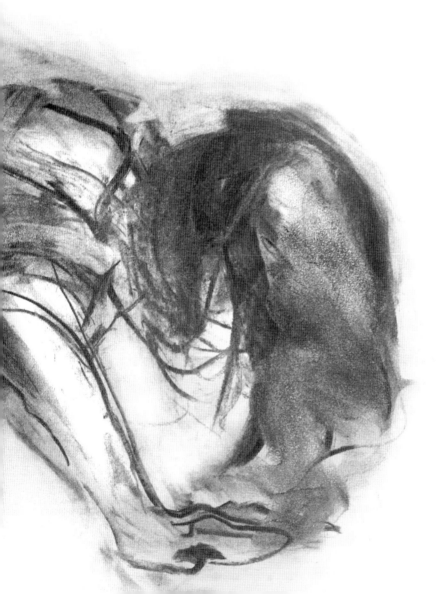

The Skeletal Experience

From Bone to Energy

We pass through varying densities and textures. We sense bone, soft tissue, fluid; we release energy and experience what might be called space or inner emptiness.

As we open up from within, as tensions resolve, insight deepens and the fog surrounding sensory appreciation begins to lift, we can feel new possibilities. Sensitivity varies between individuals. A clear, well-delineated feeling for the depth and fluidity of the lumbar spine might be enlightening for some and common place for others. There is a broad sensory scale between surface activity and the pulsatile nature of deeper areas. If someone says they can feel their spinal cord moving there may no reason to doubt it. Identifying what we feel, sensing the components of our material selves, enhances practice and brings deeper areas into focus as they become more active.

The surface of the body is rich in sensory nerve endings while deeper areas are generally less amenable to awareness. This changes as we go deeper and the spine begins to feel more alive. The work of Bonnie Bainbridge Cohen and others suggests that we can sense and work with our organs. Traditional practices suggest we can feel and influence energetic currents running through and around the spine. The conductive activity of sensory nerves may not be felt but we can feel the consequence of their sensitivity arising from the structures and organs that they serve. Sensory information presents three categories:

- sensations immediately available for perception,
- sensations that are elusive but can be made available to perception,
- sensations deemed unavailable for perception or unconscious sensory activity.

Feeling into the body presents a variety of sensations, some indicating sensory understanding at a profound level. We can feel hard tissue/bone, soft tissue, fluid, energy, space.

These components have *materialised out of each other*, bone deriving from soft tissue, soft tissue from fluid, and fluid from energy and space. Components are interdependent and *feelable*. We are reinforced by bone and moved by tissues (with nervous input), which are fed by fluid. Underlying this arrangement is the movement of energy and presence of space. All components may be felt in any combination as a *sensory cocktail*. As sensitivity awakens, we devolve. Awareness retraces the evolutionary journey, from bone to energy and space.

Feeling receptors (proprioceptive/kinesthetic) are located in muscles, connective tissue (soft tissue) and joints. Receptors for sensory stimulation to vibration and pressure are found in subcutaneous connective tissue and in the periosteal covering of bone and joint capsules.

Skin is easily felt as the sensory precursor to going inwards, followed by underlying soft tissue, the shape and orientation of bone, the depth of articular space and fluid release. We might start with the tissue having the most density, i.e. bone. Visualising bones can bring them to immediate awareness.

Deepening sensation is forthcoming when using attitudes not influenced by positions that impose tension. Primary attitudes underpin all movements and postures. Yoga postures are extensions of supination, pronation, side lying, all-fours and standing, and represent positions that we have unfolded from and into. Primary attitudes consolidate the contact points with the ground and enable the breath to find clear pathways. Primary attitudes address tension efficiently, enable a less impeded access to deeper areas and give scope for adjustment and natural expression.

If necessary, it may help to refresh anatomical visualisation through a book, model or CD ROM.

Feeling Relationships

The skeletal experience is above all else about feeling relationship. We can *sense* the shape of bones but *feel* their relationship through movement. Bony contact with the ground is a primary sensation felt through sensory nerves in the intervening tissue registering pressure. Surface bone can be felt through contact points where tissue is thin, such as elbows, knees, shins, ribs or the spinous processes of vertebrae. When we feel bone through the pressure of an outside object, such as the ground, we are touching ourselves through the agency of the object.

We can sense the shape of bones within our flesh. We can feel the skeleton through its surrounding soft tissue. Sensory nerves between tissue and bone and within the periosteal coating of bones convey a 'sense of bone'.

Sensing your skeletal framework includes feeling into your articulations. Your joints arise where their bony shape ends. We can feel the articulations as organs and as inter-bony spacers. Joints combine to provide an articular system functioning as an integrated organic unit. The skeletal framework is a sensory continuum. All joints are continuous through periosteal (around bone) tissue (fascia). Articulations are rich in sensory nerve endings, enabling us to feel the relationship, movement and rhythm between bones. With the understanding that movement creates sensation which in turn creates awareness it would seem that whatever moves has a potential for being felt.

Bones move in space during voluntary and involuntary movement. Inner activity is clearly felt when we hold back expansive movement of the limbs and spine. The deepest, most fluid movements are involuntary and are stimulated by the breath and gravitation. Involuntary movement is ideal for sensing bones and articulations. The absence of tension that arises through 'doing' gives the investing tissue more sensitivity.

Involuntary movements are stimulated by the diaphragm working with the spine and thorax. The subtle movements and rhythms of the spine can be transmitted through the limbs to the hands and feet, gradually diminishing in amplitude as they move further away from the centre.

Approach the skeletal framework by letting go of it. This enables the muscles that support and control it to reprogramme their control towards a quieter and more expansive action, an action free from gripping.

Returning the Long Bones

The long bones arrived at a later stage of evolutionary history as we pushed ourselves up and outward into our environment. They are perfect examples of growth gestures. In the womb, the limbs are held close to their central axis. Following birth, babies tend to hold their long bones close to their spinal centre, as their deeper body consolidates strength and orientation, enabling the limbs to unfold from the spine as growth and movement progress. When we use the long bones as levers, as in expansive stretches, they work against the spine as opposed to working with it. Long bones complement or work against spinal expression.

The four corners of the trunk contain sockets for the femoral and humeral heads. These joints are well lubricated for free rotatory and universal movements, giving their long bones plenty of scope for adjustment and angle changes in relation to the spinal axis.

We can feel the integration of the arms and legs with the spine through the shoulder and pelvic girdles. The girdles act as conduits, transferring action between limbs and spine and protecting it from mechanical stresses. All long bones meet through the spine and thorax, and it can feel as if the arms are rooted in the pelvis and the femurs in the shoulders. The long bones also rotate internally and externally with the breath.

The long arm bones behave in the same way as the thighs but more so because of the lightness and design of the shoulder girdle in relation to the thorax, spine and head. The arms stimulate the thoracic spine through the shoulder blades and create more space within the thorax for breathing. Returning the arms to the spine assists its potential for lengthening through its long axis and stimulates an integrated action of the spinal curves.

The thigh bones extend upward from the knees and into the pelvis at an angle through the neck of the femurs and femoral heads. They turn inwards like a large pair of bony tongs that hold the pelvis from the sides — this action can be used in practice as a supporting element for the pelvis and enables the sacrum and tail to move forward.

The sacrum represents the back of the pelvis and the spinal base. The thigh bones are attracted to the spine through the pelvis and at the sacroiliac joints. This attraction can be enhanced by gently drawing the legs back into the hip joints. Due to their soft tissue connections, the femurs may feel as if they come up into the sides of the spine as far the diaphragm, the angle of the ribs and the shoulders. This sensation follows the natural tendency of the long bones to give themselves back to their point of origin along the spine. Drawing the femurs back to the spine stimulates the lumbar and dorsal curves.

Pelvic Sensation

Your pelvis is more than a girdle. It is influenced by, and influences, everything above and below it, from the hands to the feet, including the head and jaw, and is intimately connected to the breathing movements of the diaphragm and thorax.

Your pelvis is an organ in its own right. The first thing to feel may be its weight. It contains fluid, organs and deep muscles, and the bones are heavy in their living organic state. Pelvic perceptibility deepens practice — you can go right inside your pelvis. Your pelvis and spine have evolved as a mobile unit. Working with and through the pelvis enhances the vitality of the spinal curves. Feel the long femurs returning to the spine through an organic pelvis. The fifth lumbar ver-

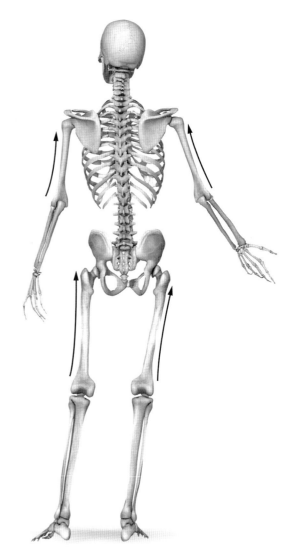

Figure 11.1

Drawing the long bones back to the spine.

tebra and femoral heads can be included as immediate aspects of the pelvis due to their articular relationship.

You can sense pelvic shape, texture, heaviness, lightness, organic nature, pulsatile power of expression and at times its emptiness.

You can sense your pelvic bones in all positions but can *feel* them directly through their prominent contact points with the ground which are easily felt and provide ample *resting down* areas for gravitation. Depending on your position, gravity may pass through the sacrum — the side of the hip bone — the front of the ilia, and on occasion the pubic bone.

Movement between the bones are easily felt as you breathe, apart from the pubic joint which has hardly any movement and acts as a springy buffer. Movement can be felt between the fifth lumbar vertebra and sacrum, between the sacrum and large flared hip bones (ilia) and between the lower pelvis and heads of the thigh bones. The whole pelvis moves from the hips and lumbar spine and the sacrum moves between the ilia.

The sacroiliac (SI) joints are feelable because they move, but are generally mobile in women and have a tendency to fuse in older males. They are only capable of small movements, but we can feel their amplitude grow as the system opens up. They are extremely responsive to deep work and their activity can be felt in the spine, shoulders, jaw and down through the legs, ankles and feet (Figure 11.2).

We may spend considerable time on the sacrum. Locally, the sacrum provides a spinal base and a back for the pelvis but its relationships are extensive. Due to their axial location, respiratory rhythm is greater at the sacrum and SI joints than at the pelvis as a whole. We may eventually visualise and feel the front of the sacrum in its continuity with the front of the spine.

The sacrum is said to float between the ilia. This may be difficult to appreciate by the more mechanically minded until it is felt. It is also suggested that the fifth lumbar vertebra is suspended between the ilia and floats between the other lumbar vertebrae and the sacrum. These suggestions are realised when practice reaches the *floating stage*. It may feel as if the entire spine and sacrum float in a fluid medium. Respiratory movements are greater at the sacroiliac joints than at the hip and pubic joints; i.e. axial respiratory movement is greater than appendicular respiratory movement.

The pelvis is naturally tilted down at the front and up at the back. This tilt is essential for producing the lumbar curve above. On rare occasions there may be a forward slipping tendency of the fifth lumbar vertebra forward on its sacral base. In such cases or when the lumbar curve is unduly exaggerated, it is helpful to follow the large hook-like movement of the tail bone on exhalation. It is also helpful to open out the lumbar curve by lying face up and dropping it into gravity — engage the front of the spine on the out-breath and pause. In standing, when the slip is vulnerable, releasing the lumbo-sacral joint by dropping the sacrum creates more space for the fifth lumbar vertebra without disturbing the function of the curves and the relationship to the femurs. Work from the front of the spine, engage the deep hip flexors, and abdominal muscles as they follow the diaphragm, the entire mechanism

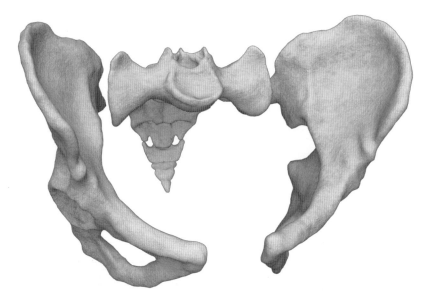

Figure 11.2

A visual sense of sacro-iliac spatiality and a floating sacrum.

working as a unit to lift the pelvic floor and drive the tail upward.

The pelvis is more sensitive when initially disengaged from the spinal base and hip joints. It also helps to *undo everything above*, from the jaw, shoulders, upper to lower spine and to release tensions in the rib cage in order to let go of the pelvis completely. Once the pelvis is free, the movements that pass through it are freer. You can then feed your legs into your pelvis to make space throughout the entire skeletal system. It helps to disengage the pelvis in order for a subsequent deeper engagement on the next exhale.

The osteopathic centre of gravity is at the body of the third lumbar vertebra but others site this centre at just in front of the sacrum at the second fused segment. When the pelvis is free and suspended from the spine, you can feel the connection between both centres as an imaginary gravity line passes through them. This sensation involves the depth of the lumbar spine and the hollowness of the pelvis. As we evolved on to two legs, the gravity centre may have played between the S2 and L3.

When standing, the pelvis receives the upward thrust from the ground but is also *suspended from the spine*. Can you let go of your pelvis and sustain the letting go? Hang your pelvis from your spine — give it away, disown it. The habit of holding on to the pelvis might be so well established that we may not be able to facilitate this for more than a moment or two. Letting go of your pelvis involves freeing it at the lumbo-sacral and hip joints. Abandoning the pelvis and not regripping it involves giving yourself and your conditioning away. When we let go of all the negative tension in and around the pelvis for more than a few moments at a time, we cultivate and sustain a new way of relating to it. The pelvis is prepared to receive deep action from above and below. We are more grounded on all levels.

A Tail

The tail bone is an extension of the spine and also belongs to the pelvis due to its location and its supportive and rhythmic action within the pelvic floor. The human tail normally reaches a maximum length of one-tenth that of the embryo in the fifth embryonic week,

and disappears during the next 3 or 4 weeks by regression, cell death and by the rapid increase in the size of the buttock region. At term, the coccyx represents the tail remnant. Some newborns display an extended tail which is soft and easily removed (England 1983). Some teachers, given a choice at that stage, may have opted to keep their tails; such can be the emphasis on tailbone activity in practice.

When you look at the tail in the adult, it is extensive and longer than imagined, resembling a large hook-like

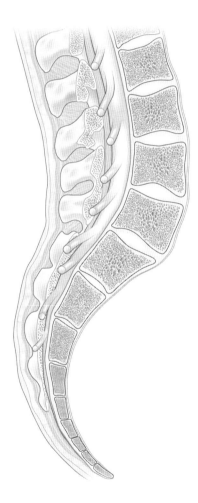

Figure 11.3

The tail is a dynamic respiratory hook. We can feel its action influencing the entire body in all postures and movements.

pointer for the entire spine above. It moves substantially with the breath when the system above is free and when the body is well integrated. We can sense the front of the tail and its continuity with the front of the sacrum. The tail works most efficiently when it is *taken along by the rest of the system and the breath.* Consciously tucking it under is a local movement that creates tensional patterns around the pelvis and disconnects from the rest of the body. Your spine ends and begins at the tip of you tail. Flexion and extension of the tail in breathing are important movements to the release and action of the body as a whole.

From Axis to Digit

> *The spine gathers and moves its appendages as an integral expression of its power.*

The large limb articulations are connected to the deep body. The ankles, hips, knees, wrists, elbows and shoulders are feelable connections to the spine. Working the arches and palms, (arches of the hands), the fingers and toes stimulates the depth body. Encouraging ankle and wrist space and digital engagement with the ground engages the spine and stimulates the diaphragm in any position.

Keeping the elbows and knees slightly flexed enables a rhythmic engaging relationship between the centre and the periphery. The base of the large and lesser toe is internally and externally continuous with the deep arch of the foot and ankle. This relationship influences everything above. As the arch lifts *an open, active space moves into all the articulations from ankle to skull.* The power of involuntary activity engages the entire body from axis to digit and back again.

Each foot has 24 bones with 32 joints between them. It might be worth reviewing their relationship, particularly the position of the cuboid and navicular (see Figure 11.4C) and the length of the heel bone as it extends forward into the arch. The arch of the working foot is well known for its roles in supporting the spine, influencing the confluence of spinal curves, and also in assisting the pelvic and thoracic diaphragms. The relevance of the contact points between the ground and foot in practice is well established, particularly at the heel and the base of the large and little toes. The length of the heel is of particular interest as it extends upward from its contact point with the ground, taking up almost half of the length of the main body of the foot (see Figure 11.4B). The front of the heel is lifted into the main arch from below by work going on locally and also through the ankle and leg. Arch space, ankle space, knee space and hip space extend upwards through the spine and into the jaw. These spaces are mutually and rhythmically interactive and supportive (Figure 11.4A). The hand – wrist relationship to the spine is also relevant. On or

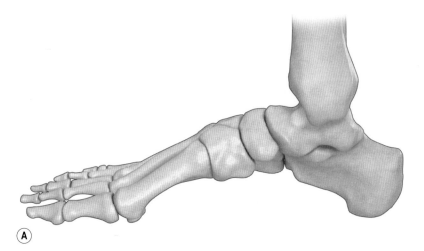

Figure 11.4A

The action and feel of the simple bony medial arch of the foot mechanically influences everything above. Its potentially powerful movement supports and opens all articulations from the ankle to the skull.

(A)

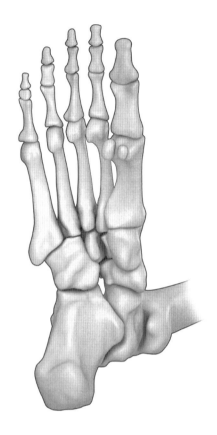

(B)

Figure 11.4B

The heel bone takes up almost half the length of the main body of the foot. The front of the heel bone lifts to become an integral part of the main arch.

off the ground, active hands and fingers stimulate the spine. The contact point between the pisiform bone (see Figure 11.4D) and the ground is particularly relevant because it opens the outside of the shoulder.

The Thorax

The inherent compliancy of the thorax accommodates and enhances all breathing and spinal movement and invites us deeply inside.

You can feel deeply inside your thorax, which, more than any other area, gives an actively spatial sensation (see Figure 11.5). A respiratory cage with the potential for rhythmic dimensional changes, thoracic activity can be felt throughout the entire body and plays an essential role in the 'depth experience'. The connective tissue lining the cage gives the feeling of drawing down into the pelvis and up into the shoulders. The thorax, diaphragm and thoracic spine can feel like an organic whole, becoming ever softer and less differentiated.

In terms of movement, the ribs are essentially breathing bones but provide an important purchase for the breath work of the diaphragm and in activating the spine. A stiff or weak thorax impacts on the spine as a whole.

You can clearly feel your ribs move in a downward wave on the in-breath and an upward wave on the out-breath. Without thinking, you can simply move with the waves of the ribs. The arrangement of the internal intercostal muscles and connective tissue lining of the interior cage is powerfully active on the exhale and during the pause.

You can experience your thorax as an elastic cage supported by fine, blade-like ribs. The inter-rib spaces, articulations with the spine, costal cartilages and absence of a frontal attachment for the lower ribs give the cage a pliability that influences the body as a whole, not only in regard to oxygenation but also mechanically.

At least four sensations arise from the ribs. These include subtle movement, strong expressive action, space and softness. The ribs gel with the spine and articulate in two places at the vertebral body and at the transverse process. At the end of the exhale, the primary cage sensation is a powerful opening from within as it works with the spine.

You can feel your thorax take an active part in the expression of the spine, head, shoulder girdle, pelvis and limbs. Rib movement is intimately tied to the shoulders and arms as the upper limb and girdles are continuous with the thorax.

The spine represents approximately one-quarter of the back of the thorax. As the thoracic spine moves inwards for the inhalation, it takes the vertebral ends of the ribs with it. This movement goes with the opening of the thorax at the front, the approximation of the shoulder blades and the widening of the collar bones at the sterno-clavicular joints. *Wait for this deep action to arrive at the end of the exhale!*

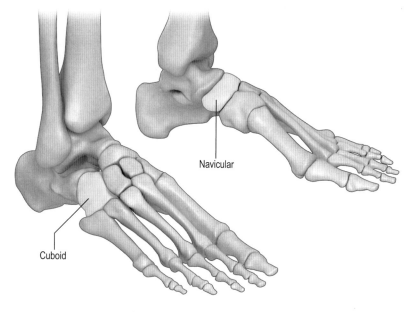

Navicular

Cuboid

Figure 11.4C

The navicular and cuboid have important roles in supporting the medial and lateral arches and are dynamically involved in directing the weight of the body away from the ground, opening all weight bearing joints and freeing and activating the thorax, shoulder and jaw. We can begin to sense these pivotal bones.

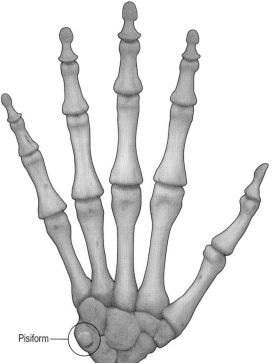

Pisiform

Figure 11.4D

The pisiform acts as a lateral heel bone to the arm as its contact to the ground activates the arch of the hand and feeds and opens the shoulder and upper spine.

Expressing Your Head

Your head is an expanded organ of expression, a continuation of your spinal column, receiving and following skeletal activity coming from below – your head and skeleton respond to each other. Your head has mushroomed out of its primary stalk, the spine.

Your head is ever-present in practice because it houses thought and sensory recognition. It also picks up the expressive power of the spine through its immediate connection with the upper cervical vertebrae. Mechanically, there is a two-way relationship between the head and spine. The head receives from the spine and also gives back to it. You can disengage your head on your neck to give back to your spine and your neck re-engages as it picks up from the spine. When organising the position of your head, these seemingly opposite movements can occur almost within the same moment.

You can feel your head, spine, diaphragm and pelvis functioning as an organic unit as they move

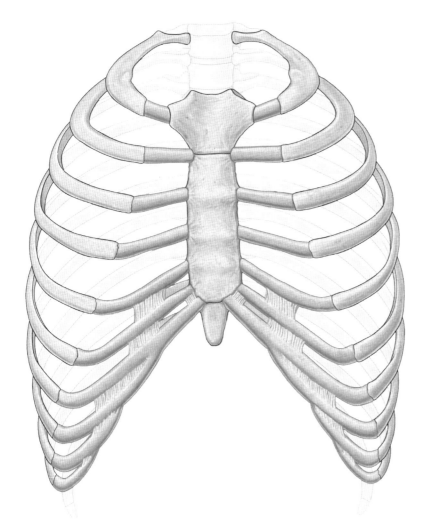

Figure 11.5

We can feel the thorax as a dynamic organ in posture work. Thoracic compliance is due to the costal cartilages, an articular relationship to the spine, the fineness of the ribs, and to the deep action of the respiratory tissue. We can use the thorax and accentuate its activity as and when necessary.

with breathing. The deep waves of the spine move up towards the head and down into the pelvis. When your spine regains its natural power, its deep action leads the head and moves it from below.

The head can be appreciated in a number of ways:

- as a top load balanced by the spinal curves,

- as a base that suspends the spine and pelvis,

- as a pointer leading the body – the skeleton follows the head,

- as an attachment for the jaw bone,

- as an attachment for the facial muscles,

- as a container for organs that feed the primary senses of balance, awareness in space, sight, hearing, taste and smell,

- as a container for organs producing cerebrospinal fluid,

- as a container for the unfolding strata of nervous tissue that has evolved from below,

- as a temple for the upper reaches of consciousness.

We can sense inside the head, stay on the outside, or have a sense of both simultaneously. In its development, the head has expanded from within outward to accommodate the evolution of the brain. The cranium is an extraordinary feat of organic engineering. The shape of its bones, the intricacy of its articulations and the structure of its internal sinuses, ridges and depressions represent a vault that has, over millennia, been fashioned by an ongoing response to its external and internal environment.

Head Bones

Your head has 22 bones made up of eight cranial bones and 14 facial bones. Cranial technicians acknowledge subtle movement of cranial and facial articulations that allow growth and the transmission of rhythm coming

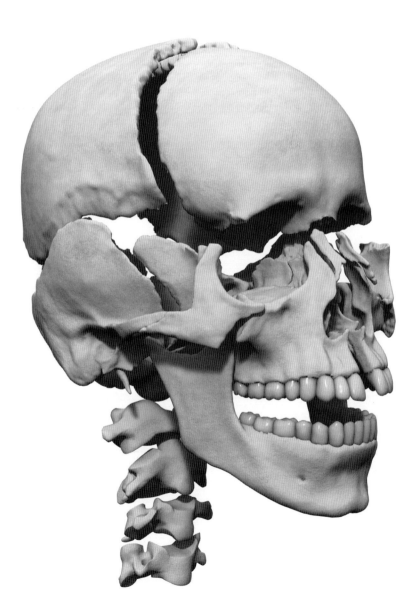

Figure 11.6A

This gross representation of the cranial bones and some of its articulations, supports, in part, the feeling of cranial expression, and a potential for experiencing subtle activity throughout the head as it picks up from the spine.

of the cranial bones and suggest that this movement is a response to cerebrospinal fluid fluctuation affecting a membranous system within the cranium.

It is thought that the brain itself is the stimulus driving a cranio-sacral system (Upledger & Vredevoogd 1983). The primary driving force may well be a combination of the fluctuating pressures of cerebrospinal fluid and the activity soft tissue elements that line the cranium internally and divide the brain compartmentally.

Cranial, spinal and sacral activity represents a continuum. A deep rhythmic activity arising into consciousness can be attributed to this continuum. It reveals itself during the more subtle aspects of practice. This involuntary motion provides an example of an original behaviour expressing itself simply because it can (with respect to its life-sustaining function) and is intimately tied to breathing and gravitation. Its enhancement is pleasurable and enlightening.

Working with the Head

Three models are generally used cranially (as with the rest of the system). The bony, soft tissue and fluid models are functionally inseparable. The fluid model is simpler because one can sense the entire skull as a soft organic fluid container. Certain cranial areas provide effective contact points with the ground and, when used, can release the neck and spine and stimulate deeper respiration through the diaphragm.

The occiput contacts the ground in supine positions. Few occiputs are symmetrical at their contact points. Further to this, muscle tension in the neck, shoulder, spine, pelvis and beyond will tend to pull more on one side than the other. Consequently, when we *give our head away* it will tend to roll to that side. As we go with the tension, the spine unwinds from above.

Rotation of the head feeds through the spine into the pelvis and influences the sacrum and sacroiliac joints. With sensitivity, we can feel head rotation through the hips, legs and feet. When the head is rotated and the pelvis lifted, the spine will bring the head back to a central position. The spine spontaneously adjusts the head – pelvis relationship.

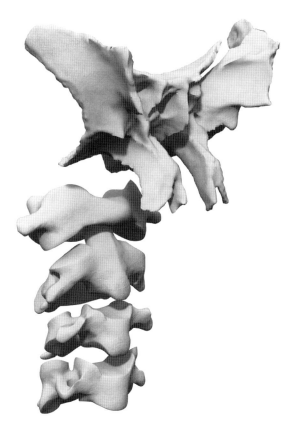

Figure 11.6B

The sphenoid is a key cranial bone. Its central position as part of the floor of the cranium, its relationship to the occiput and to the top of the spine suggests that we might feel its presence through the subtle activity of the mechanism as a whole.

from within the skull and the body below. Head and body together *embody* one interconnected organ.

The occipital bone is the largest and has a *foramen* for the passage of the spinal cord. The sphenoid, (see Figure 11.6B) so called because of its wing-like structure, is the most interesting due to its shape and function. The two bones articulate to form a large part the *floor* of the cranium. The sphenoid is central to the floor of the skull and is central to cranial mechanics and fluidity. Cranial technicians regard the sphenoid as the primary driving force for the subtle movements

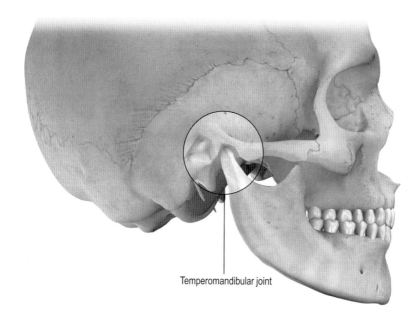

Figure 11.7

The jaw.

Temperomandibular joint

In the prone position with the head rotated, we can rest on a temporal (temple) and cheek bone, but the neck should have the flexibility to accommodate the rotation. Resting lightly on the frontal bone (forehead) for short periods may prepare the neck for a spontaneous extension as it picks up from the spine below.

The head needs monitoring to keep the spine free and to receive the activity from below. We can give the head back to the spine in small rhythmic movements. Returning the head works well with giving the shoulders and arms back to the spine. This practice of *soft shrinking* frees the thorax and spine for action, deepens the excursion of the diaphragm and assists gravitation.

Visualising the *spheniod* (Figure 11.6B) internally in resting positions may bring it to awareness. The sphenoid is a midline bone that is continuous with the front of the spine. It is known to move with the breath and has a deeply significant role in involuntary movement. We can feel the *palatine* bones by placing the tongue on the roof of the mouth. This contact appears to release tension within the cranium as a whole due to the integral relationship of all skull bones, internal and external.

In the final analysis, it is better to have *nothing in your head at all*. Have no expectation or anticipation, be empty-headed and receive the activity. Your head will express itself.

Your Jaw

Your jaw is more primitive in origin than the head as we know it. Biting existed before cerebral expansion. The jaw feels primal. When it engages, we feel like creatures about to act. The deep action of the jaw tends to repudiate thinking.

When we release the jaw, the pelvis and legs drop and we become more grounded. When we work up from the feet through the spine, the jaw engages and displays a strong and active opening from within. Its relationship to the entire body below can be dynamically felt.

The joint of the jaw presents as one well-defined articulation. We can locate the TMJ through direct contact with the fingertips when opening and closing the mandible.

During the second stage of labour, there may be an instinctive need to stretch the jaw in order to facilitate the opening of the pelvic outlet. It is also common to arch the neck and open the jaw during orgasm. You may feel a need to express your jaw during primal movement. When the jaw engages in concert with the primal activity of the spine and limbs, we appear as creatures seeking something. The spontaneous action of the jaw is a further indication of the deep interconnectivity that can be awoken and felt.

The Soft Tissue Experience

Soft tissue

Soft tissue speaks, guiding us with its sensitivity, texture and intelligence. It is the way in to primal activity.

All components of the myofascial–skeletal system that are not hard tissue (i.e. bone) can be seen as soft tissue. Soft tissue can be perceived as one organ enveloping bones and passing through articulations. We can sense soft tissue as a complete, feelable and intelligent organ in its own right. Our interest lies in the sensory properties of skin, muscle and fascia.

Soft tissue is responsive to how we are, holds our tensional patterns, and gives us our sense of self. Our soft tissue experience defines practice. Soft tissue may feel dull, tense, reactive, tired, stubborn, excited, enthusiastic, relaxed or responsive. The adjectives used to describe how we feel also describe the quality of our tissue.

Are our tissues sentient? Sentience is defined in *The Oxford English Dictionary* as 'susceptibility to sensation'. Sentience also means consciousness. Are our tissues aware of their own sensitivity, do they have such intelligence? This view is productive, as it reduces a tendency for imposing negative tension and invites us to listen closely while we work. The overall sense of tissue arises from the general activity of sensory nerves. As we practice, attention to tissues sense invites a constant flow of sensation into consciousness. The more we refine our practice, the more we feel. Our purpose is to pass through external tissue, to reveal the primal activity of the deeper layers. We experience ourselves through feeling, and the deeper we feel, the deeper the experience.

We simply tune into the quality of sensation, but the science of sensation categorises sensation as either proprioceptive, kinaesthetic, or interoceptive. Proprioceptive sensation refers to the position of body parts in space and also to balance. Proprioceptive sensors are found mainly in muscle tissue and are sensitive to contraction and stretch. They function mainly beneath consciousness. Kinaesthetic receptors are found mostly in articulations and their capsules and convey feelings of movement. Interoceptive receptors are densely distributed throughout fascial structures and provide feelings of aliveness and fine differences within soft tissues. Interoception usually referred to visceral sensations but this has now been extended to take in a wide range of sensations.

Working with Skin

The skin is appealing because we can immediately see, touch and feel it. It is the ultimate sensory organ and an open door to deeper tissues. Skin is connected by fascia to underlying muscles, bones and their articulations. Changes in skin can also illustrate the health and condition of tissues beneath it.

B.K.S. Iyengar referred to skin in the following way: 'Everything cannot be observed by our two eyes. Each pore of the skin should act like an eye. Your skin is a most sensitive guide' (Iyengar 1987).

Ashley Montagu writes in his classic *Touching, The Human Significance of the Skin*:

Perhaps next to the brain, the skin is the most important of all our organ systems. The sense most closely associated with the skin, the sense of touch, is the earliest to develop in the human embryo. When the embryo is less than an inch long from crown to rump, and less than six weeks old, light stoking of the upper lip or wings of the nose will cause bending of the neck and trunk away from the source of stimulation. ... As the most ancient and largest of the sense organs of the body, the skin enables the organism to learn about its environment. It is the medium, in all its differentiated parts, by which the external world is perceived (Montagu 1971).

The skin is *the* original tissue because all creatures, organisms and cells are bound by an enveloping skin or membrane; we are contained by skin. Montagu points out: 'There is a general embryological law which states that the earlier a function develops, the more fundamental it is likely to be' (Montagu 1971, p. 6). This statement places skin high on the list of tissues instrumental in taking us inwards. Skin and the central nervous system have unfolded from the same primal layer of tissue (ectoderm). In this regard, the brain and skin are inner and outer reflections of each other. The skin is a neurological surface projection of deep sensory centres. Sensory nerves supplying the skin are also tributaries of nerves that supply underlying muscle.

Muscle changes are picked up by the skin and can direct us to where we may need to work. Consciously appealing to the skin to open or soften has a direct effect on underlying muscle tissue and in this way influences integration and the ability of the organism to express itself. We can enter the body through the skin to locate the deeper layers of tissue. The skin also moves with the underlying superficial fascia. One of the most helpful suggestions is to move the skin covering a given area to stimulate the muscle below.

We influence the skin by internally engaging the breath and spine and move outwards towards the surface from within. The skin gives information regarding deeper activity and expresses it externally. The skin is also in contact with the space around us. As sensitivity increases, this becomes a viable sensation. The spine

and our immediate external environment converse through the mediation of the skin.

We can invite the skin to open over a given area, encouraging underlying resistance to follow suit. We can spread a localised movement over the entire surface of the body, moving from *skin to skin* and working with its fine continuous patchwork. This has a direct effect on the quality of perception. You can direct the underlying muscles and bone through the skin. For example, drawing the skin covering the top of your foot upwards and over your shin opens up ankle space and lifts the arch. Inviting the skin to soften and shrink over a given area is effective when giving back to the spine. As you give the appendages, girdles and head back to the core you can soften your skin to give the underling tissues a greater sense of release, enabling the spine to act spontaneously. These actions are driven by underlying superficial fascia connected to your skin, but it is your skin that you can see, touch and relate to.

Whether we move in a new direction or return to a familiar one, the skin, in terms of contact with the ground, the space around us, deeper activity and our general state of awareness, is a key factor in *going inwards and expressing outwards*.

'The skin is the intellect – a sense organ, flesh is physical ... all knowledge comes only from the skin' (Iyengar 1987).

Feeling Muscle

Muscle tissue is the executive organ of our body, literally the executor of our will. It is proposed that muscular activity occurs mostly beneath conscious awareness (Juhan 1987). Unconscious muscular sensation is concerned with relaying information to the nervous system regarding the positional relationship between parts of the body and to the space around us (proprioception). Sensory receptors in joint tissues are deemed more available to consciousness and give us awareness of movement (kinaesthesia). Tension receptors that belong to muscle have proven to be relatively insentient, in that we have no conscious perception of their activity. But it *feels* as if we do feel our muscles, and this appears to happen indirectly. We can also visualise muscle tissue and imagine its activity.

Deane Juhan writes: 'Yet it would be patently absurd to imagine that muscle tension and movement play no part in our conscious sensory experience' (Juhan 1987). He suggests that conscious muscular perception arises from ongoing pressures and movements of muscle tissue stimulating surrounding nervous tissue (Juhan 1987). The movement and internal contact of tissue on tissue provides a conscious sense of our muscular activity. We feel muscle indirectly through its stimulatory effect on local nervous and connective tissue. In this respect, movement is the key to conscious perception. Movement that arouses conscious sensations of muscular activity and texture can be externally provoked by the will, such as the movement of an arm, or by the internal movements of breathing while working or at rest.

Interstitial (exracellular) receptors richly innervate the fascial tissues within and around muscle tissue and are part of an 'interoceptive' system of sensory communication that is concerned with fine tuning of sensory information. These sensations target the 'insular cortex', an area deeply within the centre of the brain, but also feed the sensory cortex above (Schleip 2012).

Not only do we feel muscular tension, contraction, stretch and release, we also notice pulsations and vibrations and become sensitive to a muscular presence in and out of practice. Muscular activity, whether felt indirectly or directly, is inextricably alloyed to a culture of perceptible nervous activity. Scientific inquiry is ongoing. In time, new discoveries might well reveal other sensory possibilities. As late as the 1960s, some 'authorities' still held the view that the newborn had little if any awareness of its sensations. Around this time, some individuals were conducting their own experiential research into the effects of yoga and LSD and discovered nuances and depths of physiological experience that under normal circumstances were considered beyond awareness. Conscious muscular sensation is a fact of life and practice and might still yield an untapped potential for feelability. As we attentively refine our sensory inquiry we access new and deeper movements and connections. It is helpful to have our experience explained in physiological terms by an out-side authority, but the personal work provides the personal experience.

Deep Muscle

We have unfolded from deep central muscles. All muscles spring from a central source, but the deepest and most centralised provide power and stability. As we work, these muscles draw us inwards on exhalation, and release us outwards on inhalation. When actively engaged, they work as a unit and little if any differentiation can be felt between them. We feel the action and the area but not the individual muscles, but some muscles should be mentioned because of their central importance.

The thoracic diaphragm, pelvic floor, iliopsoas, abdominal and intervertebral muscles are key players. The inner thigh muscles, the adductors, can be felt as core muscles as they draw up from the medial arches of the feet and feed the spine on each side. The combined action of the central muscles spreads in all directions, and we can return to them with every breath.

Surface muscle is easier to feel than deeper muscle. This is because of the sensitivity and palpability of skin overlying surface muscle, but as we proceed, our deep muscles predominate in awareness and we might feel like organisms moving from an ancient place within ourselves.

Muscles are numerous and varied and, with the odd exception, are paired from the midline. Even the thoracic and pelvic diaphragms, although centrally disposed, can be felt as being two-sided. We can evaluate the relationship between each side and direct our attention to the side that needs to work harder. Muscle responds directly to our will and is sensitive to how and what we think. You can feel this when you trace negative tension back to what your mind is doing. Muscle that cannot be felt can be visualised. As deep movement comes into awareness, we can visualise and feel the tissues involved. You can visualise and sense the muscular activity of the diaphragm, the small intervertebral muscles, and the activity of all the central musculature of the body extending outward as one organ into the hands and feet.

Feeling Fascia

Muscle and fascia are functionally inseparable, hence the term *myofascial*. Muscle and nerve are inseparable hence *neuromuscular*. The term neuromyofascial can apply to feeling. Connective tissue in the form of fascia contains sensory nerves. You can feel your skin and underlying superficial fascia working together. Muscular sensations derive from fascial investment which is rich in sensory receptors that convey sensation to awareness.

Fascia works through the more active agency of the muscles but has contractile properties. The pervasiveness of fascia is well documented. It surrounds and pervades every tissue in the body. It extends over bones, invades joints, surrounds muscle fibres, organs, and thickens throughout the lower back and soles of the feet. Fascia is like a supportive, interconnecting bindweed; nothing remains untouched by it, and for this reason it has the primary connective function throughout the body.

The fascial continuum beneath the skin is easily engaged and we can work with it at will. Superficial fascia is continuous with deep fascia in and around bones and joints. It weaves its way into the recesses of the depth body, spine and diaphragm, and lines the abdominal, pelvic and thoracic cavities and invests the central muscles.

When your body pulls itself together, the action is weighted towards the fascia as a *drawing and interconnecting agent*. When you feel strength and power arising from the depth body, the sensations are more muscular but may reach consciousness via a fascial component. Lifting and opening the arches of your feet is initially muscular but the effect in your shoulders and jaw is a consequence of fascial integration.

When you activate the fascia in the palms of your hands and soles of your feet it feels like four peripheral diaphragms giving back to, and receiving from, the thoracic diaphragm, thorax and spine.

'The feeling of joint spaces opening up is probably conveyed by the fascial component of capsular ligaments' (van der Wal 2012). The inner dance of the bones coming to awareness may also have a sensory fascial component.

The fascia at the back of the waist (lumbar – dorsal fascia) and soles of the feet (plantar fascia) is particularly thick and its activity is easily felt. Actively stretching the toes activates the pelvis and diaphragm via the fascial continuum.

Fascial structures that compartmentalise the brain and surround the spinal cord are also relevant to deep action and may be considered as part of the soft tissue experience, either directly through fine tuning, or following initial visualisation and imagination.

Working Soft Tissue

Skin, muscle and fascia provide the soft tissue experience. We can focus on each tissue or on soft tissue as a whole. Fascia is the organ of connectivity, and although it carries contractile fibres, the muscles move us and do the real work. In essence, muscle and fascia are impotent without one another. During the act of practice, there is no real need to separate fascia from muscle in our sensory awareness or imagination because they function as one.

We work with soft tissue in various ways:

- Organising the limbs, girdles and head in relation to the spine involves sensing bones and articulations through soft tissues.

- The muscle that envelopes long bones moves through and around the girdles, the spine, thorax, abdomen, waist, hands, feet, fingers and toes as an *organic whole*. When we approach the system organically we can feel them working as a complete responsive system.

- Releasing the large external muscles by giving our weight to the ground and following the breath into the spine assists the small muscles of the spine, the diaphragm and the deep fascia in opening the body from within.

We can change tissue texture at will because it is responsive to mental suggestion. Suggest softness to an area and it will soften. Think soft and tissue softens, become ambitious and it tenses, think wide and it widens, think long and it lengthens, think deeply and we pass through it.

Overthinking tenses soft tissue, while lack of interest or attention sends it to sleep. We can sense the presence of tissue at rest and its aliveness when working.

Stretching tissue externally has a different effect because it imposes upon the spine's power of expression. Applying tension by drawing parts of the body away from the centre inhibits the emergence of deep involuntary activity. The spine moves from its depth when it leads movement, i.e. when the long bones are centred. This impetus sets up a deep and powerful unwinding that involves fascia, muscle, and moves out to the skin. As disengagement proceeds and we alternate work with softness, the differentiation between skin, muscle and fascia dissolves. One organ, one action.

B.K.S. Iyengar, well known for his role in bringing yoga to the West, made a science of stretching. His contribution to this end is immeasurable. He went to 'great lengths' in trying to adapt Western bodies to an approach well suited to Indian/Asian ones.* Many of his students have gone on to modify, adapt and refine his approach, often going in different directions through their own exhaustive inquiry. Vanda Scaravelli is a case in point, and in her own way made a science of *undoing the body* by making the fullest possible use of the ground and the breath. Feldenkrais, Alexander Technique, Tai chi, Chi- Quong and classic osteopathy are just a few examples of activities that manage well without pulling on muscles and provoking resistance.[1]

Within the total soft tissue arrangement, muscle provides the most resistance and sense of release in practice (unless there is a joint fixation). If our intention is to bring the body towards an original state, we must court the muscles, respect their sensitivity, and treat them as a representation of the deeper intelligence that resides within us. But muscle action cannot be deepened and integrated without simultaneously attending to its fascial investment and covering layer of skin.

Does it Matter?

When we are feeling deeply and completely, does it matter what route sensation takes or which of the soft tissues are involved? Is it necessary to identify the various structures taking part in a total organic rhythm? In one way, it does matter. We should know our working material, its shape and its relationships. Dividing sensory experience into components is helpful, if only to put them together again. Iyengar identified more than 150 workable areas on the skin, with the understanding that they were connected. The analytical exercise is worthwhile if it stimulates interest, and if interest stimulates feeling. The words kinaesthesia and proprioception are useful if they clarify our experience. It can only help to know *what* we are feeling, and *how* we are feeling it. We can then allow the names of muscles and the nature of fascia to roll by. We can pass through sensory categorisation and move on. But we may need to identify a new or deeper sensation through anatomical reference. On one level, external information feeds into our sensory system, but on another level we move through and beyond all the information and its detail. At its simplest, tissue sensation guides us as it flows inward and upward to register in the sensory brain. Once we feel tissue as a totality, what next? We can go more deeply, fostering fluid and spatial sensations as they arise, as energy moves us.

[1]*Apparently there is no word in Sanskrit for stretch, but there is for expansion.

The Fluid Experience

We Are Fluid

A feeling arises that can only be described as a fluid release. Tissues dissolve and bones float as sensations of liquidity take us beyond anatomical differentiation. Ideas regarding fascia and muscle are absorbed by waves and our experience tells us that fluidity is an original state.

The fluid feel features in various styles of work. When tension recedes and we move *beyond structure*, we may feel like a fluid organism bound by a membrane, the skin. As we decondense, our fluid component flows freely. This experience may touch a memory of an embryonic environment and fluid origin. At eight weeks in the womb, we are nearly all fluid, in life we are 85 per cent water. The fluid feeling, when prolific, appears to signify a return to a developmental stage before gravity condensed our tissues, moulded our bones and established the neuromuscular reflexes that support us on land. In practice, we might experience fluidity as a deep surge rising towards the skin and then falling back to repeat itself for the next involuntary movement of inhalation.

Fluidisation involves a total change in texture. We feel seductive sensations under the skin, within the articulations, throughout soft tissues and around the bones. This all-encompassing experience has the effect of washing away the habitual self and its complexities. Where does this feeling come from; is it a fluid release or just a softening of tissues, or both? Are sensory nerves picking up feelings of fluid production, release

or circulation? Is fluid waiting in the wings to release itself and, if so, where does it wait? Do we produce more fluid in practice? Perhaps fluid is like consciousness; the slightest change feels substantial in comparison to our habitual state. Are we dry without knowing it?

Fluid is Fluid

Fluid is categorised into blood, lymph, interstitial, intracellular, extracellular and cerebrospinal fluid (CSF). To us, it *feels like one fluid*. If fluidity is an original state, there must be an *original fluid* (salinity). We experience fluidity as a tidal expression grounded in an original undifferentiated state.

Sensations of deep fluid movement are possibly driven by the CFS, which has engaged the imagination of many therapists and teachers. It is of particular interest because of its depth and function. CFS acts as a shock absorber, protecting and 'buoying' the brain and spinal cord, enabling them to float within the skull and vertebral column. CFS filters nutrients from the blood to the central nervous system and removes waste and toxic substances.

CSF is produced within the deep cavities of the brain by a process of filtration and secretions from networks of capillaries. CSF runs down and around the spinal cord, tracking through spinal nerves within fascial planes to the rest of the body. It blends with interstitial fluid before being reabsorbed by the venous system. CSF moves down the back and up the front of the spinal cord as it circulates. The direction of this flow compliments or is complemented by the 'up the front and down the back' suggestions made by some postural re-educators, notably Mabel Todd.

Exponents of the Fluid Body

Fluidisation is a consequence of practice, but may not be a direct focus. We are initially busy with skeletal and soft tissue sensations and tend to look to others more directly *immersed* in the 'fluid field' to shed light on what might be behind our fluid experience.

Theodor Schwenk, a pioneer in water research and founder of the Institute for Flow Science, describes our fluid origins. He states: 'Developing forms of life arise from a fluid base. Every living creature, in the act of bringing forth its visible shape out of its archetypal idea, passes through a liquid phase' (Schwenk 1962).

Emilie Conrad, the author of *Life on Land*, developed an approach to health focused exclusively on the fluid body. With a background in dance and through her inspired work on herself, she founded the movement therapy Continuum. Emilie Conrad lived the fluid life. She writes:

As I become more adept at consciously entering into the fluid system of my own bodily tissues, I experience my fluid self as a kaleidoscope of all species – their features and adaptabilities, their forms and functions. The fluid within our bodies recapitulates its own history along with the archaic wisdom of cellular heritage. When one can merge consciousness with this fluid, a completely different order of existence emerges (Conrad 2007).

Andrew Taylor Still, the founder of osteopathy, wrote as long ago as 1892:

We continue our investigation, but the results are not satisfactory and another leaf is opened and the question appears, why and where is the mystery, what quality and element of force and vitality has been withheld? A thought strikes him that the cerebrospinal fluid is one of the highest known elements that are contained in the body, and unless the brain furnishes this fluid in abundance, a disabled condition of the body will remain. He who is able to reason will see that this great river of life must be tapped and the withering field irrigated at one, or the harvest of health be forever lost (Still 1902).

On my first meeting with Vanda Scaravelli, a remarkable and inspiring yoga teacher, she asked me about cerebrospinal fluid. She told me she had resolved an elbow problem and that in her opinion it had been the fluid release arising from her breathing practice that had a healing effect. I explained my understanding of CSF, which appeared to make sense to her.

Fluid Feeling

The fluid feeling is fluid moving. Breath and fluid move together inside us. The breathing wave stimulates the fluid wave and the fluid wave invites the breathing wave. When you wait, inside yourself, within your deep waist, when the exhalation has disappeared inside you, to a place where you cannot follow, an inner lake with infinite depth, you may feel pulses, delicate adjustments and nuances of *something*. It might be the movement of blood through the major vessels and their tributaries, or a rebalancing of your diaphragm and associate tissues, or deep eddies of CSF, exploring its environment. These involuntary physiologically orchestrated movements possibly indicate a sensitive cooperation between CSF, the delicate activity of the diaphragm, quiet muscular activity, and the motion of the spinal cord and brain.

Fluid will take the path of least resistance, and to promote its flow we must open impeding physiological and psychological resistance. Fluidity becomes more prolific as tension dissolves. Reaching into the involuntary action of the spine and the deepening action of the breath reveals a fluid tendency that wants to happen. All categories of fluid, in whatever combination, present themselves to the forefront of awareness as one pulsatile, wave-like, enlightening entity.

Fascial structures within the skull, spinal column and limbs possibly influence CSF flow by way of a reciprocal tension that extends throughout all connective tissue in the body. Cranial practitioners suggest that this mechanism supports and drives 'primary respiration', an activity that underpins respiration as we know it, and that it provides the fundamental life supporting process.

Practitioners working with reciprocal tension influence the involuntary movement related to CSF fluctuation by working with the movements and rhythms of connective tissue, fascial planes and the mobility of the cranial bones and sacrum. In our practice of working on ourselves, we create these responses by refining the breath and our attention. During the quieter aspects of practice, free from voluntary interference, and when sensitive enough, we can feel a fluid movement drawing the breath. We can feel a tide attracting respiration from within. When practice is more demonstrative, when it takes off during more active movements, we feel like the fluid organisms we are, undulating, activating, moving through the skeletal structure and its tissues.

Moving from Fluid

The way we move influences the degree to which fluid release and flow takes place. Wave-like spiral movements articulate bones and joints and free the mechanical body from holding patterns. These movements, coupled with respiratory rhythms, stimulate a fluid release which in turn enhances the quality of mechanical movements. The mechanical and organic aspects of our original nature inform each other. If fluid release is stimulated by practice, we can safely assume that the breath stimulating the spine, spinal motion stimulating the breath, the alternating engagement and release of fascial planes and muscle activity, a movement of the cord within the spinal canal and a calming of mental activity, combine to produce a fluid effusion and production. The activity of the body, essentially its involuntary component, stimulates fluid release.

In nature, flowing water contains patterns of fine, delicate movements. Water not only flows downward, following the path of least resistance, but also revolves around its own flow. The organism begins to form through vortices which are spiral. We get a sense of this when we are quietly attentive before an inhalation. The spine is internally and externally bathed by fluid, and when invited, it moves sideways, front to back and back to front and rotates in combinations of waves and spirals. Birth involves a spiral emergence of the infant

and one of our first movements following birth involves rotation. Osteopathic mechanics point out the integral relationship between rotation and side-bending in the spine. We can feel the potential subtlety of this relationship, particularly when a quiet practice follows a more stimulating one. As we lie on our backs and breathe, we can detect subtle rotatory and sideways movements of the spine as it floats in its fluid environment. Theodor Schwenk writes:

It is not possible to speak of the beginning or end of a circulatory system, everything is inwardly connected and reciprocally related. ... let us recall that water endeavours to round itself off into a sphere, to become an image of the whole cosmos. If a directional force is added to this, for instance the force of gravity, then the combination of the two – sphere and directional force – will result in a screw-like or spiralling form (Schwenk 1962).

Schwenk points out that the directional structure of bone is testament to the movement of fluid expressing itself in the musculoskeletal system:

An examination of joint formation in man and animal shows that the fine spongy bone structures in the ends of bones runs straight towards the surfaces of the joint and continues on the other side of the gap as if there were no interruption. Even solid bones solidify originally out of a liquid state (Schwenk 1962).

We are also supported by fluid. Bodies of water exact a force against gravity and the fluid element of the human body, in some measure, provides a resistance to gravitational pull, bringing a sense of lightness to our work.

Sensitivity and Fluidity

As we become more fluid, we become more sensitive. Fluid is the food of sensory nerves. The sensory system thrives on vascularisation, CSF and lymph. Fluid release and rhythm feed our ability to feel the fine differences and nuances that arise during deep work. Our fluid base delivers intelligence to our sensory system, enabling a release of tension, an integrated action, and reduces the possibility of strain.

There are times when we translate into a sensory, amorphous, pulsating organism, devoid of structure and structured thought. We reduce to a sensorium, free from mental registrations and recognitions. Fluidisation cleans the slate. We move into the state described as pure awareness, sensitivity free from content. Schwenk writes:

Even in water the surfaces of the forms that are created are unbelievably sensitive. It is a sensitivity that is not based on any nervous system but arises out of the interplay of forces and is not to be understood from the aspect of the material. How delicate then must be a skin that constitutes a boundary surface which is also differentiated in material! Surely here nature reveals one of its secrets by anticipating sensitivity in flowing movement without needing a nervous system! Does it not actually incorporate in the material of the nerve-sense organs in living creatures the sensitivity already present as a function in fluids? ... The form of the jelly fish is no more than an expression of the simple pulsating movement in a source, transformed through the resistance of the surrounding water (Schwenk 1962).

The fluid state does not divide or belong in one particular place but is everywhere at once. Fluidity is continuous; it does not have the resistance of bone, tissue tension or ideas.

Fluid Body – Fluid Self

Sensations of fluidity in the body also fluidise the self. Definitions of fluidity describe ways of being that we aspire to in life. Easy, natural, unbroken, graceful, elegant and rhythmic are among those definitions denoting that we feel good. *Being fluid* is also defined as *articulate*, which can apply to our articulations. Our freely movable joints are indeed full of (synovial) fluid. The term also implies *expressive, communicative, coherent, cogent* and *illuminating.* When we feel fluid we feel free, flowing, smooth, effortless, uninterrupted, adaptable and open to change. We can take our pick. The point is that the fluid-self embraces desirable qualities.

Fluid, meaning to flow, comes from *fluent*, from the old French *fluie*, meaning *stream of our conscious state.* Eastern disciplines describe 'a *stream* of consciousness'. Consciousness has arisen out of a fluid base. Through the body we can tune into the fluidity that lies beneath our conditioning. Thought may be fluid; the mind in meditation may be fluid. Spiritual guides describe the potential stillness of the mind as being a movement without the disturbance of thought.

As we find ourselves in the fluidity of practice, ideas about fluidity become redundant. Ideas, although useful as in initial tool, are another form of resistance. Ideas are essential for progress but impede the flow of organic continuance. When we are *in fluid*, an idea, a stiffness of the mind, can be as much an impediment as a fixation between spinal vertebrae. The difference is that, when you see the idea, it can be dropped in a moment; the spinal impediment takes longer.

As the fluid body opens up to *what is*, so does the fluid mind. We move into a state of de-condensation, free from the density of habit. When we fluidise we let go of individuality and gel with those around us. Fluidising groups have a remarkable quality of integration, non-invasiveness and compassion. Immersed in an organic process, a fluid group has nothing to say, think or aim at. It moves as an expression of life — because it can.

Returning to Fluid

Returning to fluidity is transformative but we must work for it. The way in follows the practices so far. Touching the spine with the breath, yielding to gravity, myofascial release and engagement, centring bones, working with the respiratory and movement capabilities of the diaphragm, the rhythm of the sacrum and tail bone stimulate a profuse fluidity. Any turn of practice that de-condenses negative tension and appeals to involuntary expression will appeal to our fluid physiology.

At the end of or during practice, lie on your back and drop the end of your exhalation into your fluid centre and leave it there. Feel the ripples extend outward throughout your entire system — allow it to happen. As the fluid expands there may be an inhalation waiting in the wings — it will arrive — but perhaps not yet. The inhalation will be guided by the expansion, the breath follows the fluid. Give your long bones back to your fluid base. Disappear into the end of your exhalation, and immerse your consciousness into deep liquidity.

Fluidity occurs in any position or transition from pose to pose, whether working at a slow or a faster pace. Working more actively in postures and switching from pose to pose involves being awake enough to catch the fluidising release for the in-breath to arrive. The movement of the tail bone in concert with the breath enhances fluid release.

The movement of fluid has given us form, and the continuation of movement within form is constantly present. In this respect, there is no such thing as stillness. Stillness is relative. Involuntary movement can feel more alive and active than its voluntary counterpart. If life is an expression of itself, life's basic expression is the movement, waves and pulsations of fluid.

The earliest embryonic cells thrive and unfold within a culture of fluidity and softness. Our ability to harness power from our environment stems from a most vulnerable beginning. It is an extraordinary thing that all our technology, creativity, destructive and constructive tendencies arise from the delicate union of a sperm and egg cell within a culture of fluid. Our machinery, great buildings, scientific genius, art, achievements, abilities, aggression, stupidity, intelligence and capacity for love, everything that we are and might be, arise from a fluid base. Organic practice explores a return to a liquid origin that underpins our totality. We can start again, with the possibility that our more positive aspects will resurface and predominate.

The Energy Experience

The Fact of Energy

The energy experience takes us a subtle step further. Sensations can be profound. Energy is the currency of existence, it radiates from the deepest centres to well beyond the surface of the body.

Energy is the fact of life, an invisible fabric of activity around which all physiological and psychological functions occur. All experience, consciousness, subconsciousness, activity and tension is energy. We are condensations of energy and have evolved from an energy base. As we decondense, release tension, gravitate, open and move from our centre, this base reveals itself as a sensory experience. We *are* energy, and we wake up to a deeper energetic feel as the deeper body awakens. Both science and Eastern practice have contributed to our understanding of energy. Energy is unseen but we see its manifestation in living flesh and everything around us. Energy is a vast subject commanding the interest of physics, quantum mechanics, healers, yogis and martial arts exponents.

We are told that body energy is made up of electrical, magnetic, elastic, kinetic, gravitational, thermal and chemical energy. Various energies are said to arise from organs and systems. For example, liver energy may pulse at a different frequency than heart energy. Energy condenses to form structures but is always moving. Bone, soft tissue and fluid are manifestations of energy and also conduct it. The soft tissues and fluids are well suited for conducting energy. Energy is a potency waiting in the wings.

The 'energies' must have sprung from a common source. James Oschman, a pioneer into the nature of energetic healing and author of several books on energy, notably *Energy Medicine*, points out that Albert Einstein spent the last decades of his life in an unsuccessful search to find a common denominator behind the various forms of energy as a totality. Oschman acknowledges that, at a fundamental level, science is unclear what energy actually is (Oschman 2000). The yogis had no problem with energy, and felt it as a unified phenomenon that blended personal and universal sensations. If we accept ourselves as the sum of all energies, as 'organic energetic units', we can acknowledge and sense energy on this level.

The Experience of Energy

We *are* energy. The more we *feel ourselves* the more energised we are. Increased feeling indicates we are releasing more energy. We feel energy moving through the agency of sensory material. To be felt, energy must pass through substance. Energy is sensed because it has a consciously alive pathway to pass through. Energy awakens within the tissue it consists of, and is its own host, passing through a condensation of itself.

All sensation can be attributed to the movement of energy. For centuries yogis, martial artists and healers have been masters at tuning into this phenomenon. Tapping into primal currents and vibrations, and sensing the connection to the energy rich space around us may be a familiar experience for some of us. If one is an energy sceptic, you only have to relate energy to tension.

The greater the tension in a given area, the greater the condensation of energy needed to sustain it. Releasing the diaphragm can be followed by deep and powerful energetic sensations. Equating energy with tension experientially invites distinctions. Deep body energy may feel different from surface energy. The disruptive energy of mental interference feels at odds with the energetic feel of pure attention. The impediments highlighted in Chapter 8 are based on energetic disturbance and also spend energy. The tension of expectation, non-essential thought and ambition use energy, and impede energetic flow. The release of tension that comes from silence, effortless gravitation and the emancipation of the spine enable energy to move freely, feeding the body-mind on all levels. The external muscles, when excessively tense, withhold energy from the deep body. When the body is in harmony, the deep and superficial body exchange and share energy. The energy of a teacher's voice may help or hinder group work.

Practice enhances feeling, and deep work deepens feelings that can be described as energetic. The energy experience is variable. Sensations include aliveness, tingling, heat, vibration and radiation. Energy is carried by and also produces vibrations, pulsations and waves and can include subtle to strong sensations of streaming. These feelings have the same organic origin, i.e. basic biophysical energy (the life force), presenting itself where needed and as the opportunity arises, usually in dormant areas.

Aliveness is a general energetic feeling in the background or foreground of awareness. When quiet, following practice, you may feel like an organic tuning fork humming with vibration. Feelings of 'aliveness' indicate that energy is 'on the move' and gives a heightened sense of self. We may feel the finest sensations as micropulsations or microwaves.

The energetic sensations produced by *decondensing* can move upwards, downwards, towards and away from the centre, circulating, through the spine, tissues and skin. We may feel energy moving up the front of the body and down the back, up one side of the spine and down the other. Because thought influences sensation, you can *think energy* in any direction. For this reason it is more useful to allow energy to happen as a consequence of the general work. Feelings of general aliveness and vibrational activity are free to spread and do their job of revitalising the organism.

Primal Energy

Form and consciousness are the products of organic energy with its origin in environmental energy. Organic energy is *the* primal movement. James Oschman agrees with the Eastern idea of 'one energy'. He writes: 'Early on in the embryo there is no nervous system but the cells are there as a consequence of the primal energy that constitutes all' (Oschman 2000).

Mechanical, fluid and energetic waves are connected. The mechanical wave of the spine is the most accessible, whether stimulated by gravitational response, breathing or both. When we find the mechanical spinal wave, we stimulate the fluid and energetic waves arising from a deeper level. When we pare back to primal activity in ourselves, it becomes clear that the deep body is an energetic powerhouse. The mechanical wave action of the spine is tied to its energetic properties. The ligaments, muscles and fascia of the deep body produce elastic energy. The spinal fluid carries energy in its flow, and the spinal nerves conduct energy to and from the rest of the body. The entire arrangement feeds awareness and our sense of self. We may not feel the distinction between these activities, but by cultivating the feeling of waves we invite sensations that can be called energetic.

'Mechanical waves, such as those produced by the cranio-sacral system, the beating of the heart, the breath and "muscle sounds" will give rise to electromechanical waves that spread throughout the living matrix. ... Moreover, the whole body is polarised, with the head end negative and the tail — or foot — end positive' (Oschman 2000).

Tissue and Energy

Energy touches tissue as it passes through it, and needs the tissue's substance and sensory aspect to register its movement. We do not need to think about moving energy but can focus on its manifestation as a tissue sense. We can feel in ourselves how every breath, pause and movement of a spinal bone releases and creates energy. Each time we let go of thought, we release energy. 'The activation of specific processes goes hand in hand with opening of the channels for the flow of energy and information. The free flow of messages through tissues is essential for – simply feeling well' (Oschman (2000).

A.T. Still, the founder of osteopathy in the late 1800s, and also regarded as a magnetic healer, knew that reorganising the tissues had a vital energetic effect in healing. Ida Rolf asked 'Is "balancing" actually the placing of the body of flesh upon an energy pattern that activates it. The pattern of this fine energy would not be as easily disorganised and might well survive relatively intact' (Rolf 1977). She suggests that energy may be an activity around which all physiological functions occur.

'Virtually all of the tissues of the body generate electricity when they are compressed or stretched. The piezoelectric effect is partly responsible for these electric fields. Another source of such fields is a phenomenon known as streaming potentials' (Oschman 2000). Wilhelm Reich referred to sensations of energy release as 'streamings', resulting from freeing the breath, pelvis, diaphragm and abdomen.

The connective tissue fabric also conducts bioelectricity between every part of the body. Each movement generates bioelectric activities that are characteristic of the tension and compressions of the movements. 'The underlying reality pattern is once again one of energy currents, energy interplays — energy transfers from less dense to more dense media and back again. Muscular expansions and contractions foster these transfers' (Rolf 1977). Perceiving ourselves as condensations of energy includes the realisation that we have an energetic hub, i.e. energy from the spine and its contents radiates through us and beyond the surface of the body. This is our experience, what we feel following deep integrated work.

Energy East and West

Eastern and Western energy are the same energy, the fundamental difference being that the East needed no proof of energy; they felt it. The yoga masters manipulated their energetic discoveries in order to reveal the mysteries of the universe in relation to consciousness.

They came to the same conclusion as Western science many centuries later — everything is energy and is connected by energy. For millennia, Eastern practitioners understood, felt and worked with the fact that we are condensations of energy. Energy has been the staple diet of Eastern practice for many centuries.

Eastern practitioners had no problem with depth; they went into themselves and kept going. The traditional yoga practitioners developed an experiential science out of energy movement. They tuned into energetic circuits and currents that are basic to life. In this sense, yoga reveals primal activity. The yogis decondensed their body-minds and worked with the energies they discovered at a deeper level. Their approach in relation to ours in the West is well put by Elmer Green in his foreword to John Upledger's and Jon Vredevoogd's book, *Cranial-Sacral Therapy*. He writes: 'I am especially struck by the many parallels between the sensings and manipulations in Upledger's "direction of energy" and the sensings and manipulations of "body electricity" in yogic theory and practice, both in yogic intervention and in yogic self-regulation' (Upledger & Vredevoogd 1983).

He continues: 'According to classic yogic theory, the body's neurological network is a correlate, or reflection, of a more primary network of "nadis", which are filaments of super-physical but real, substance not yet detected by instruments. These filaments are constructed, it is said, of "dense prana", and they conduct a more subtle form of prana throughout the physical structure.' Green's observations are well known to yoga practitioners.

You cannot directly *do* energy and although the yogis appeared to manipulate energy with a precise reference to energy centres and channels, they arrived at a system of energy work through an indirect application of breath work, meditation and mental focus. They worked through substance to reach the energetic experience.

Our own experience may detect energetic currents through the limbs, over the skin or trunk. We may feel energy moving, from the centre to the surface and back again. We may experience ourselves as transmitters, each of us conducting and radiating energy, and connecting with others within the same field. We share radiation with one another other and collectively with the energetic field of the planet. Each person is a plexus connecting with neighbouring and distal plexuses and the deeper we go into the body the more we awaken as a total radiating unit of energy. It appears that meditation and yoga enhance the kind of consciousness that enables brain waves to become entrained with the micropulsations of the earth's energetic field.

Plexuses, organs, articulations, tissues and brains are said to have varying radiations. The heart is said to radiate at least 15 feet (detectably) away from the body (Oschman 2000). Some individuals may have a greater radiance. It's not uncommon in a workshop to open arms, radiate from your deep chest and feel the energy come back through the back of you as if it is circumventing the globe. We may also contain energy and keep it circulating within for a 'yoga high'.

The yogis followed their energy release upwards to an alternative consciousness. Westerners have always had an interest in this concept. Ida Rolf writes:

... it is noteworthy that the physical techniques of yoga were not indulged in merely for their own sake for exercise. Their practice, together with the control of breath, was a means of stimulating the nervous emotional system in such a way that, among other changes in consciousness, the phenomenon called Kundalini could be evoked. Development of this kind of energy, especially through breath control, brings out another aspect of human personality, normally latent in our time – the psychic (Rolf 1977).

The Kundalini experience could be described as an energetic emergence of primal activity revealing itself in the absence of personal patterning.

Energy and Fluid

The circulatory system is a primary channel for the flow of energy through the body:

It is a basic law in physics that when an electric current flows through a conductor, a magnetic field is created in the surrounding space. Pulsations and waves indicate that fluid flow charged with energy is releasing throughout the system.

... Molecules do not have to touch each other to interact. Energy can flow through the electromagnetic field. The electromagnetic field, along with water, forms the matrix of life. Water can form structures that transmit energy (Oschman quoting Szent-Gyorgi 1988) (Oschman 2000).

In our practice when fluid release is profuse and we lie down, focused on pulsation and lubrication, we can experience a heightened sense of vibration throughout the entire organism.

Wilhelm Reich, in *Character Analysis*, discusses how he works beneath individual patterns, going beyond the physiology of nerves and muscles and focuses on the organism itself. Physiological and psychological functions are 'taken up' by the organic work. He was interested in the biological 'core' of the organism, reflected by the *plasma system*. He points out that: 'the most primitive and most advanced plasmatic function exists side by side and function as if they were connected to one another' (Reich 1942). Reich focused on biological energy transmitted in wave movements and wave-like pulsations and used the term *orgone* to denote organic energy. He acknowledged that living material derives from non-living material and non-living material derives from cosmic energy; i.e. we are made of universal constituents. Emilie Conrad, a leading exponent of fluid practice, continually cites the essential role of fluid in energy conduction in her book *Life on Land* (Conrad 2007).

Mechanical Factors and Energy

Mechanical health is related to energy conduction and economy. Classical osteopaths and others see joints as conductors or pathways of energetic flow. Vital energy is said to course through healthy and *open* articulations and nerve impulses conducting sensory motor pathways are known to flow unimpeded through joints free from stress and misalignment. Muscular balance, postural freedom and ease of movement are the outward indications that supportive energy passes through the system with minimum impediment. This implies a good working relationship between bones at their joints, particularly spinal joints, but also at every joint because of their interactive relationship.

Yoga has always recognised the spine as the energetic and mechanical centre of the body, and that attending to the spine mechanically is a primary factor in releasing its inherent energy. As practitioners, working on ourselves and in groups, we have no doubt that energy flows more freely when articulations are open, and the bones perform their inner dance. Oschman writes:

In terms of the magnetic fluxes through the vertebral column and surrounding tissues which give rise to the overall field of the body, the best arrangement is one in which the axes of the fibres are parallel and in alignment. Departures from the parallel arrangement will tend to reduce the total magnetic flux through the system and thereby reduce the overall field. In other words when the spine is in alignment and free from bending and other imposed stresses the energy can flow freely and powerfully (Oschman 2000).

He further states: 'A consequence of this point of view is that every joint in the body participates in the energy flow essential to life and that alignment depends on both the position of the hard tissues (bone) and the arrangement of the surrounding soft tissues (ligaments and tendons).' This statement by Oschman (2000) resonates with classic osteopathic practice and yoga, and confirms the relevance of working *from the spine* as opposed to imposing the limbs and their girdles upon it. When the spines expression is unimpeded, its associate energy flows freely.

Gravity and Energy

Physics states that each of us is an energy field and the product of the larger gravitational energy field of the earth. It is accepted by many practitioners that a well-aligned body receives and transmits energy more effectively than a body holding tension through habitual misalignment. You cannot delve into the potential of gravitation without being spontaneously drawn into the tension—energy relationship. It takes tension, and therefore energy, to hold the body out of its gravity line. Reorganising the body

within its own gravitational field and the gravitational field of the earth frees energy by freeing tension.

Yoga practitioners usually have a well-established relationship with the ground. Dropping into and focusing on contact points releases gravitational energy upwards, opens the articulations and frees the tissues for energetic release. Although structural alignment is important, we can go beyond it. Our original nature produces energy beyond cortical direction and postural alignment. When the spine moves according to its own rules, alignment as an imposed factor can be inhibitive. The snake-like movement of the spine in any position indicates a mechanical freedom and powerful behaviour that releases energy.

An Original Energy System

An alternative, more ancient energy system underlying the classic nervous system has been proposed and may be an enabling factor in energy conduction and primal movement. Oschman points out:

Perineural cells surround each neuron in the brain, and follow every peripheral nerve to its destination. The perineural connective tissue generates slower-moving waves that flow throughout the organism, affecting every part. This system, unlike the classic system, does not have specific point-to-point targets. The classic system in terms of evolution and phylogeny is a relatively recent innovation. But the perineural system is a global system that integrates and regulates messages to every part of the organism. In terms of evolution and phylogeny, the perineural system is ancient. This system is responsible for the overall regulation of the classic nervous system. The perineural system is involved in several important phenomena, not least of which is the production of the hypnotic state, and the effects of geomagnetic fields on brain waves and therefore behaviour and biological rhythms (Oschman 2000).

He cites Yoshio Manaka (Manaka 1995), a leading scientist/acupuncturist, who suggests there are many 'unknown' communication circuits. He posits a *'primitive regulatory system'* that is different from the classic nervous system, one that arose in evolution long before the nervous system. It is present in single-celled animals, which do not have nerves per se, but react to external stimuli. The body's energy fields, perineural system, and living matrix are cited as the conduits that channel biocircuits. This primitive form of energy conduction supports the experience that something intelligent and beyond ourselves is at work, and that we have been instrumental in revealing it.

One Energy One Cosmos

Although Einstein could not identify it, and science cannot find out what energy actually is, it feels as if we are energy fields within an energy field. When we are sensitive to it, our experience tells us we are individual condensations of energy connected by the energy in space and the energetic pull of the earth. Body and mind are the same energy. The meridians and chakras as proposed by acupuncture and yoga might be derivatives of one total energy. The spine, heart, anger, love and politics spring from one energy base.

The experiences we have of dissolving, in which we 'feel one with everything', the microcosm blending with the macrocosm, are energetic experiences and were touched on by Wilhelm Reich and his student, Alexander Lowen (who went on to pioneer bioenergetics). They used energy release to resolve psychic conflict and acknowledged one energy in the body and its connection to the cosmos. Reich termed biological energy 'the orgone', suggesting that: 'Cosmic orgone energy functions in the living organism as a specific biological energy' (Reich 1933).

Lowen writes:

We must follow the physical law that all energy is interchangeable and we must assume, in harmony with modern doctrines in physics, that all forms of energy can be and eventually will be reduced to a common denominator. It is not important at this point to know the final form of this

basic energy. We work with the hypothesis that there is one fundamental energy in the human body whether it manifests itself in psychic phenomena or in somatic motion. This energy we call simply 'bio-energy' (Lowen 1958).

Lowen relates the flow of energy to personal strength: 'The feeling of strength depends upon the surge of life force or energy' (Lowen 1958). This is not a muscular strength referred to by Lowen, but a life affirming, assertive strength, a way of being in life that is supported by robust energetic flow. We all have the experience of energy coursing through us unimpeded, and of the overall effect it has on our way of being. A background sense of 'aliveness' has the same effect.

Reich and Lowen proposed that all energy had two interconnected functions: sexuality/reproduction and a biophysical need for organic expression. The need for expression applied to the emotions as well as the biophysiology, as emotion was seen as a 'plasmatic movement'. They proposed that energy was conducted by the fluid of the body, essentially the plasma. Reich connected plasma movement to two basic forms of expression: pleasure which involved an outward movement from the periphery to the skin, and non-pleasure, involving an inward movement. The therapeutic goal was to mobilise blocks in the muscular armouring of their patients which would enable a release of tension and energetic flow that inhibited the free expression of emotion contained in the block. Depending upon their history, clients were as likely to inhibit pleasurable sensation as they were unpleasurable sensation. Biophysical inhibitions were not only personally impairing but also acted as an inhibitive factor affecting a universal awareness of the 'bigger picture'. These ideas and the practices that support them are very much in line with the philosophical aspects of yoga. A fundamental difference between yoga and bioenergetics is that the former (traditionally) manipulates, directs and contains organic energy while the latter releases it. Reich writes:

Cosmic orgone energy functions in the living organism as specific biological energy. As such it governs the entire organism. ... What moves in this process is nothing but orgone energy, which is contained in the body fluids. Accordingly, the mobilisation of

plasmatic currents and emotions in the organism is identical
with the mobilisation of orgone energy (Reich 1933).

Oschman, commenting on the cosmic aspect, says: 'The fields within the human body are inevitably affected by the larger fields of the earth and other celestial bodies. The mechanisms are not mystical or obscure; they involve well-documented pathways of interaction' (Oschman 2000).

The point is that the organism has an inherent energetic need for expression and that this expression is non-verbal, has a language of its own, is potentially pleasurable and is connected to the bigger picture.

Relating to Energy

Does the fact that we know about energy lead us to believe it is energy we feel. If we had no knowledge of energy, we might simply interpret our finer sensations as movements springing from a common source, notably the spine, the skin and anything in between. Finer sensations of currents and streamings may arise from the classic or the perineural nervous system, or from fluids stimulating the sensory system. But we know that every cell is driven by energy and that all activity is energetic. On this basis, there is no problem referring to all experience as energetic.

Energy is movement, whether raising an arm, pulsating, vibrating, or surfing awareness. Movement also creates energy and promotes its circulation. Involuntary movements are effective in circulating energy because they undo tension on a deeper level and release fluid containing energy. Energy is an involuntary phenomenon; we can set things up to release and direct energy but it we cannot do energy because we are energy. You cannot *do* yourself. Standard physics suggests that energy is the primary force in nature from which all inorganic and organic matter, all life, has sprung in one form or another. Raw energy may or may not be channelled by a grand design. We may experience an 'energetic intelligence' that feels larger than we are, but the point is we are part of one energy.

The energy used for thought may either enhance or inhibit sensory experience. We could view the mind as a leech, sucking the energy from the body. When psychic energy flows freely it flows into the body; when physiological energy flows freely it flows into the mind. Freeing energy from the lower back is an all-encompassing experience. Energy is released in the form of heat. Heat in the spine is a common sensation, or the hands, or anywhere, the entire body can radiate heat from within. This is not the heat of warming up in faster practices – it is the heat energy from the deep centre of the body. We can feel a substantial release of energy as a result of working with the spine and deep respiratory muscles, and feel it spread throughout the entire system.

How we experience energy may influence how we practise, but how we practise is essentially the key to energetic experience. Habit can be seen as an energetic stasis. This is why it is important to explore oneself in different ways within ones practice. Our awareness of energy is also energy, and how we use our awareness can help or hinder our progress. Energy has produced a life force of tremendous power; the point is how we use it.

The energetic experience is personal, whether we feel energy through the spine, limbs or an energetic connection to the space around us and beyond. We feel it in groups. The fields of two adjacent organisms will interact with each other. 'When electric currents flow through tissues, the laws of physics dictate that magnetic fields must be created in the surrounding region. Energy fields around the body [biomagnetic fields] spread way beyond the body, indefinitely' (Oschman 2000). We all feel group energy when working with others. Fields of personal energy cross over and it's common to make deeper progress in groups than when we practise alone. Sometimes the group energy can be so strong it feels as if the surrounding space is thick and alive with it. One of the most rewarding features of group work is that we share and benefit from each other's energy.

A Word on Space

Energy inhabits space and, as practice progresses, it is common to experience sensations of 'empty space' within the body. These sensations indicate a deep release of tension as your spine, thorax and pelvis begin to open up. We are told by physical science that we are

99 per cent space. 'Early electron microscopy confirmed that cells contain substantial amounts of empty space' (Oschman 2000). Jaap van der Wal points out that in the first embryonic week only the dimension of space is present. He also views body cavities as activities; they are active (van der Wal 2003). It makes sense that we might feel space as a consequence of the tensegrity mechanism, as the long bones push out from the spine, and as the vertebral discs open up.

The thorax, waist and pelvis may feel like one continuous space, the bones feeling light as all organs of separation open up. A welcome sensation of emptiness informs us that our practice has released tension on a deep level. We may have a clear sensation of connecting to the space around us, as if our density has dissolved and we realise a spatial origin, a time before the oceans formed and we were simply energy in space. Sensing an enhanced relationship to the space around us might, in part, be due to an awakening of our skin; we have unfolded from space and feel one with it once more.

We cannot *do* energy or space, as they are a consequence of deep, rhythmic work surfacing to awareness. In whatever way we interpret spatial sensations, they signify an integrative practice. As the deep movements of the spine connect to the entire body, as bone, soft tissue, fluid and energy coalesce, merging textures, we become internally lighter: 'we de-condense. The two-week-old embryo has a ventral and dorsal aspect – nothing in the middle – it is empty. The first gesture of the evolving middle layer is to draw towards the centre!' (van der Wal 2003).

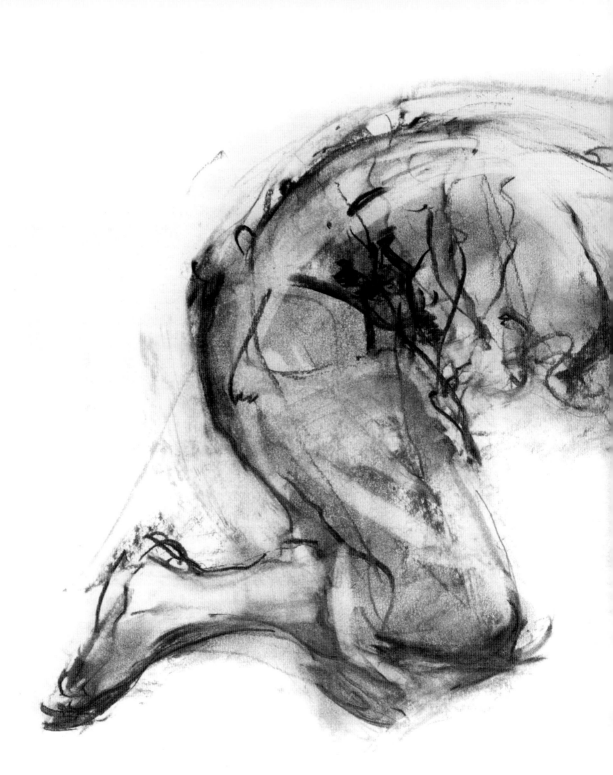

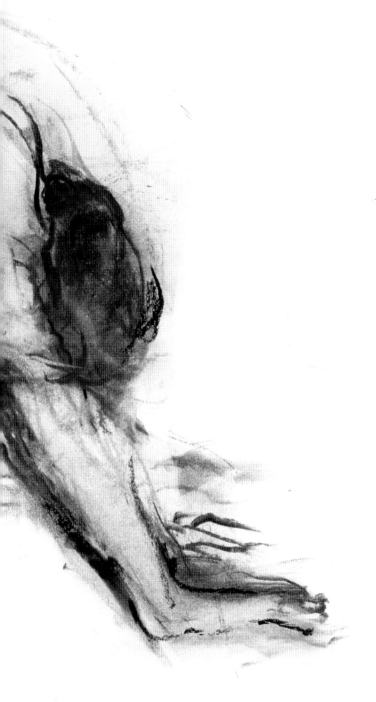

SECTION 3

The Original Spine

Centrepiece

The spine is the original body. We are classified as vertebrates. Everything we are is associated with the spine. Our organs, tissues and systems are connected to the spine and its contents. Consciousness, and all it brings, is an energetic result of spinal activity. We are an outward expression of the spine, having literally flowered from this stem of primal origination.

Eastern disciplines have long acknowledged the spine as the primary physical feature in health and personal development, and the spine gives classical osteopathy its central focus. Arousing spinal activity lays bare its primitive power, and highlights it as the physiological determinant in all practice.

As we conduct our experiential research, we discover that the vertebral column delivers a sensory experience that underpins all postures and movements. The original spine provides the centrepiece for practice and is the primary motivator that speaks from within and drives the body. We may be attracted to the soft tissues, the limbs and the fluid dynamic of the body as a whole, but the spine gives a definitive focus. Sensations arising from the hips, pelvis and shoulders are external compared to the depth of feeling arising from the spine.

Cultivating an efficient spine requires courting its sensitivity. Stretching, bending and twisting certainly encourage greater feeling, but do not guarantee the realisation of a sensory potential that comes from awakening and integrating each vertebral segment. As superfluous

tension and postural habit resolve, and we feel the spine feeling itself more deeply, we begin to recognise it as a force in its own right. An original spine is freely active and responsive with a moment-to-moment ability to inform us of its needs. It has no interest in the imposition of postures but leads us into them. The spine has vital mechanical properties but can also be experienced as an organ in its own right, within the organism as a whole.

All spines share common weak spots where the curves change and where more naturally flexible areas meet areas that are naturally more rigid. These points are found: (See Figure 15.1)

C
• where the fifth lumbar vertebra meets the sacrum,

B
• where the lumbar and thoracic curves meet at the first lumbar and twelfth thoracic vertebrae, as the entire weight of the upper body is received at this point, which is an elusive area to sense in practice,

A
• where the upper thoracic vertebra meets the flexible lower cervical area,

G
• where the top of the neck meets the base of the skull around the second cervical vertebra. It is worth noting that the atlas acts as a simple washer or buffer during movements between the neck and skull.

The centre of the spinal curves, where bending occurs more easily, are also vulnerable to weakness and strain. Bending tends to occur more easily just above and below the third lumbar, the seventh thoracic and third cervical vertebrae. See Figure 15.1 points F, E, D respectively.

Any spinal area may be prone to weakness, instability or strain. When the spine rediscovers its inherent fluidity and enjoys an articular coherence throughout, all intervertebral segments take part in an overall rhythm that reduc-

es potential strain, articulates the spine as an integrated mobile unit, and enhances and enriches all practice.

Sensitivity and good spinal mechanics feed each other. This implies that all vertebrae engage in postures without strain, that the natural spinal curves share a working confluence, that gravitational responses are clear and uninhibited and that spinal — respiratory muscles work as a unit.

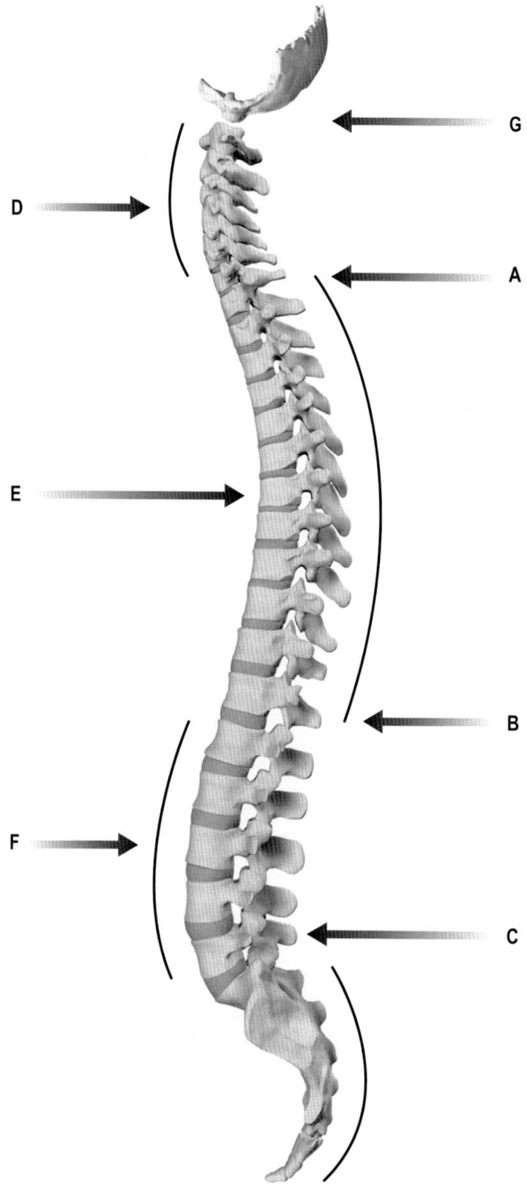

Feeling the Spine

Spinal interest is driven by *sensory curiosity*. The anatomy is useful because of the spine's primal nature, central importance, its susceptibility to strain, and its capacity for profound change. Some aspects are easily felt, others may be potentially felt, while some may never be felt. Cultivating a deeper understanding of the spine through anatomical focus informs practice and teaching.

The following points are relevant to spinal interest:

• The design and nature of the spine is the consequence of our evolution to the upright posture. As we unfolded from the ground, the spine became the centre from which all movement and gravitation occurs.

• The spine is deeply set, is pyramidal in shape, larger at the base and tapering towards the head (Figure 15.2).

• The spine is the most profusely jointed structure in the body with 120 articulations – this includes its connections to the ribs (Figure 15.3).

• The spine is a suspensory as well as a weight-bearing mechanism, suspended from the head, jaw and, by every vertebra, successively from above down. The spine suspends the pelvis and legs.

• Gravity lines pass through the spine at certain points.

• The upward thrust from the ground can be used to release and open the spine.

• The arrangement of four opposing spinal curves includes two primary and two secondary curves. They enable the spine to support the head as a top load, and, with the assistance of discs and soft tissues, give the spine its quality as a responsive universal spring.

Figure 15.1

Weak spots.

- Our centre of gravity is located at the middle of the lumbar curve and provides the opening from which all deep posture work takes place.

- Each vertebral complex presents a mobile, supportive and sensitive unit that is functionally inseparable from its immediate and distal neighbours. In this respect, all vertebrae should participate in every posture equally within their functional capacity.

- Integrated spinal mobility is dependent on the health and quality of the discs, which form approximately one-quarter of total spinal length. It is not unusual for practitioner/teachers to incur a disc injury as a consequence of limited awareness.

- The cervical and lumbar curves are due almost entirely to the shape of the discs, are more mobile and therefore easier to feel. The dorsal curve is due predominately to the shape of the bones, is less mobile and less easily felt.

- The curves have the potential for mutual rhythmic integration, and with the rest of the body. This is the determining factor in primal movement.

- The middle of the dorsal and lumbar curves relate to the shoulder and pelvic girdles, respectively, and to their long bones.

- The articular facet joints control the degree and range of spinal movement. Their capsular coverings have sensory nerve endings but it is debatable how much of their activity is amenable to awareness.

- The spine and diaphragm are intimately connected, each influencing the functional quality of the other.

- The tailbone represents a large hook rising up into the pelvic floor; it is capable of substantial respiratory motion and is an essential factor in spinal dynamics.

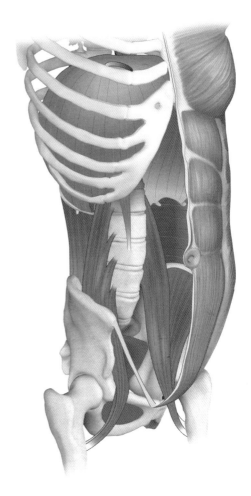

Figure 15.2

Sensing the depth of the lumbar spine.

Developmental Factors in Practice

Each intervertebral segment, as an individual unit, is capable of the spine's universal movements. Forward, backward, side bending and rotation can occur between any two vertebrae and in a variety of combinations. The degree of each movement in a given area depends upon the shape of the facets in that area. For example, rotation is limited in the lumbar spine but freer in the thoracic and cervical spine. Backward bending in the thoracic spine is limited compared to that of the lumbar and cervical areas.

We may easily feel our spine bending and extending, but may less easily feel a dynamic confluence between the curves. For example, the thoracic spine may impose stress on the lumbar spine while bending backwards or rotating. This will inhibit rhythmic communication between curves.

Small local intervertebral movements are the most important ones. When we begin to sense the individual vertebrae moving in concert with the whole spine, we have reached a higher degree of spinal intelligence and

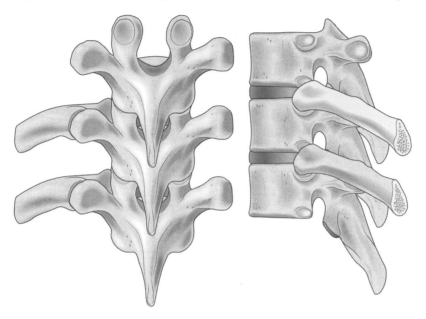

Figure 15.3A

The articular relationship between the ribs and the spine enhance spinal feel-ability.

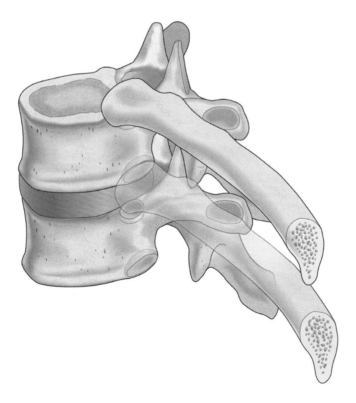

Figure 15.3B

The ribs and spine.

sensitivity. We can visualise and sense a more refined spinal action when we intentionally hold ourselves back from extending into larger ranges of movement.

When we hold back, and sense into the spine, there is little possibility of creating a lack of communication between its parts. We may perceive our spine as a collection of bones connected by soft tissues or as bones set in tissue. Bones are pre-formed in cartilage and arise out of a softer medium. When the finer activity of spinal segments feeds into our perception of the curves, and into bending generally, the quality of movement has a completely different feel. There may be a point at which the spine is so alive and sensitive that bending may appear superfluous and unnecessary, as it can inhibit intersegmental rhythm.

When we cultivate a harmonious *felt* action between all vertebrae we are providing the areas where the curves change, the centre of the curves and any bone in the spine that may lack rhythm, with an opportunity to take part in the dance and intelligence of the spine as an integrated organ in its own right.

Spinal Sensation

The depth of spinal sensation is dependent on the condition of its sensory nerves. We cannot *do* depth sensation but we can set things up for it to arise. The spine is rich in sensory nerves; some function beneath our level of awareness and some provide us with spinal awareness. The spine can feel like a muscular snake with its own autonomy. It's as if the long bones, although an essential aspect of our evolutionary development, if not used intelligently, do us no service at all, in that they exert mechanical stress and often strain through the spine, particularly at its weakest links. This easily happens when we inadvertently work against the spine. The limbs are long levers and can be used to our advantage or not.

Serge Gracovetsky, author of *The Spinal Engine*, writes:

To this day gait analysis is essentially the analysis of the motion of the legs. The legs are certainly useful, but are they essential? The answer is definitely no. Human bipedal gait will be demonstrated not to require the presence of any extremities. In retrospect, it was evident that the primary function of the spine, so evident in fish, was never transferred to any of our extremities (Gracovetsky 1989).

Spinal sensation may arise from a number of areas. The areas rich in sensory nerve endings, usually operating beneath a conscious level also have the potential for informing awareness. Sensors within the small intervertebral muscles, the investing spinal fascia, the roots of the diaphragm, the ligaments, and the articular joint capsules, may collectively provide us with feeling. As intervertebral movement increases, spinal feeling increases. As feeling increases, integrated mobility increases because we can work directly with the awakened sections of the spine.

Information not related to an actual physical experience also contributes to our understanding of the spinal mechanism. For example we may not have a direct or complete physical sense of the bony shape of the vertebrae or the ligaments, but visualising them may contribute to a deeper understanding, and sense of spinal activity, and give substance to the more valid spinal sensations.

In practice we should *feel all relevant spinal action*. But activity that is available for perception is often inhibited by tension. Tension may be habitual, or imposed by positions that inhibit spinal rhythm. We are usually unaware that our spine is unaware until it wakes up.

Aspects Regarding the Practicing Spine

- The spine is rich in sensory nerve endings.

- It has the potential to move by itself when stimulated by gravitational reflexes, respiratory and thoracic movements and appropriate stimulation from the long bones.

- The lumbar and cervical curves are (at first) more amenable to suggestion than the dorsal curve and take sensory precedence in practice.

- The lumbar curve is the most powerful, its dynamic action potentially dominating the entire body and spreading out to the limbs.

- The tail bone is an active recipient and stimulator of spinal activity.

Spinal Changes

The spine's versatility and intelligence gives it the potential for profound change. Small changes may occur rapidly and are ever deepening. Their totality over time can be profound.

Experience suggests a greater:

- spinal awareness,

- flow between curves,

- opening of disc space,

- spinal elongation,*

- space between the ribs,

- integration between the spine, girdles and limbs,

- integration between spinal and respiratory muscles,

- awareness of the spine as an organ of respiration,

- softening of the spine,

- release of fluid,

- inner strength,

- contact with the ground,

- understanding of the significance of the tail bone,

- spontaneous spinal expression,

- intervertebral movement at each segment exhibiting a more profound involuntary activity throughout the entire column.

*The spine cannot lengthen indefinitely; its involuntary nature involves retraction as it prepares for the next elongation.

The term 'central mechanism' avoids lengthy repetition in reference to the arrangement of the deep lumbar spine, sacrum, coccyx and diaphragm, abdominal, belly band accessory respiratory muscles, pelvic floor and the small muscles running between the vertebrae, in short, all the structures and tissues between and including the pelvic and thoracic diaphragms that are instrumental in deep organic movement.

Spinal Work

This section presents two basic attitudes and could be repeated from Figure 16.2 and Figure 10.3D. The attitudes are not relaxation (although one's mind is relaxed); they provide a basic framework for releasing firstly the external muscles, and then the deeper smaller ones, in order to access their dynamic possibility.

To maximise progress, let go of the idea that the spine is *your property*. Spinal intelligence existed long before the advent of the cerebral cortex and its need for identity. An approach based on ownership inhibits spontaneous movement. Perceive your spine as a separate entity, unattached to, and unaffected by, your wants or expectations.

Begin by noticing how you are on all levels. Tune into your mood, expectations, tension levels, rate of thought, and the quality of your general way of being. 'Noticing' is the foundation for all practice and should be used right from the beginning as *soon as you lie down*. Thought is not attention. Attention involves being attentive to thought, as well as to sensory information. Once relevant thought has taken you where you need to be, you can begin to let go of 'thought words' and allow 'thought feelings' (conscious registration of sensations) to take precedence:

- Give your weight freely to the ground.

- Visualise and then follow the shape of the spine. You can easily feel its contact with the ground. Activate the arches of your feet and ankles.

- Mentally assist the spine to soften and disengage.

- Using your breath as an active feeler, move into your spinal bones and articulations.

- Keep tuning into your body weight as it falls through your contact points with the ground, i.e. sacrum, dorsal spine, elbows, heels, forefoot and head.

- Soften your awareness, your inner voice, your eyes and your facial muscles.

- There is only one nervous system; 'softening' these aspects has the effect of softening the entire system, which in turn renders us more sensitive and awake.

- Your weight is still going down, down, down: gravity is a movement in time with time.

- Surrender your knowledge and get out of your own way; abandon yourself with awareness.

- Lift your pelvis slightly and place it down immediately and gently. You will notice that after the weight has released into the ground it is still going down; the weight of the pelvis is still going down and as you give it your attention it is still going down. Gravity is constant; we are in perpetual downward motion, falling to earth without pause. This may be obvious, but has real meaning when we feel it and use it to good effect.

- Your lumbar curve will have less contact with the ground and will move between flexion and extension as you breathe.

- Feel the spine freeing itself from the grip of the large muscles.

- Notice that your pelvis is still going down!

- Direct your attention deeply into the spine as it begins to awaken.

- Be creative. Creativity means 'exploring', not 'knowing' what comes next, and working with it when it arrives.

- Continue to visualise and sense the central mechanism.

- As you exhale, feel the belly band muscles suck back and up as they follow gravity and the diaphragm. Wait longer for the inhalation; it will come by itself. This action is exaggerated and continuous during the pause.

- Release the jaw by separating your lips and teeth. Your jaw can potentially engage and open in direct response of the action coming up from the spine below.

- The jaw and pelvis are dynamically connected through the spine.

- Now, work more actively to open your feet and ankles; draw up into your legs, pelvis and spine.

- Slightly, and softly, shorten the back of your neck, adopting what might be a primordial attitude, a creature-like feel.

- Exhale into your spine.

- Keep releasing your jaw. Feel your long bones come back into the upper and lower spine. The deep action comes as you are waiting for the inhale to arrive.

- Focus on your tail bone and feel its primal nature; its movement can be profuse and enlightening.

- The dorsal spine may actively soften and move with the breath.

- Imagine yourself as a primal creature washed up on the beach, adjusting to the land and receiving oxygen from the space around you; let the breath and spine move you from within.

- Tune in to the dynamic action of your coccyx and sacrum as they tuck on the exhale and release back on the inhale — exhalation is spinal flexion, inhalation is spinal extension.

- Tune into intervertebral activity: key areas such as the L5 and L3 vertebrae, the T11 and T12 vertebrae, the middle of the thoracic curve as it softens and articulates itself in relation to the ground it rests upon. Sense the front of these vertebrae from within.

- The body begins to move by itself — from the spine and then out into the arms and legs.

The alternate arm positions modify their relationship to the spine and release it in alternative ways. This also keeps the process interesting by varying the location and the quality of sensations.

As you feel your deep centre open up, you are separating through the middle of the lumbar curve, above and below the third lumbar vertebra (L3). Your centre of gravity is responding to the roots of the diaphragm at the end of the exhalation. This movement spreads throughout the entire spine down into the legs and feet and up into the shoulders, arms, head and jaw. It *is one integrative movement* and reinforces contact with the ground.

Most importantly, explore inside yourself and let sensory information guide you. It will inspire you to act, or not, as the spine reveals itself. As your spinal centre is nourished, you might be drawn into untapped and powerfully active recesses of yourself.

Involuntary Waves

We are wave-like in nature. Waves hark back to our earliest stages of development: fluid waves, the waves of labour and birth. Orgasm is wave-like, sound comes in waves, sensation comes in waves, we experience waves of emotion and brain activity is wave-like. Surrendering is wave-like as we let go, return to the action of the spine, and then let go again as the physiology takes over.

The nature of the 'original spine' is demonstrated by its wave-like reflexive nature. It moves *by itself* in an involuntary wave-like response to its environment. This feature of spinal behaviour is one of the most enlightening of all physiological experiences.

The spinal curves are wave-like in design, but when impotent, appear as a 'frozen wave'. Involuntary waves are suppressed by conditioning and habit. The alignment of vertebrae is relevant to a point, but releasing the reflexive wave demonstrates true freedom and autonomy. A crooked spine may exhibit more freedom and spontaneous action than a straight one. A spine may be well organised vertically, but also contain an inherent tension that inhibits its primal nature.

The waves are a simple reversal of the curves and a return to normal in one flowing movement. This feels like a reptilian awakening and cuts through ideas about methods, styles of working and how to *do* the practice. The waves free us from the grip of neo-cortical activity, wiping the physiological and psychological slate clean. There are no frills when this action predominates.

Working the Wave

The wave-like quality depends on a balance between disengagement and engagement. The relationship between doing and undoing is transient, and at any given moment feeling will dictate the need to pick up the action or let go of it. The spine leads and we go to meet it. Spinal power comes from awakening its nature, not from reinforcing tension in the large external muscles. The true wave is a representation of the true self, as we are immersed in an original activity.

When free from tension, the larger muscles are able to sense a deeper level of activity and also become primary sensors. Feeling proceeds from inside out and from outside in.

Smaller waves can be felt within the larger ones. They are due to the release of negative tension within the central mechanism and its subsequent response.

Subtle, pulsatile waves can be felt when the breath lies quietly between exhale and inhale. These pulsations relate to the fluid elements of the deep spine. The fluid experience arises as the bones and articulations consolidate an intelligent relationship. Their awakening underpins, and results from, the larger more muscular waves.

On occasion the spine can be felt to translate sideways – a sidewinder – you may feel a preference to one side – we all have a scoliosis. Just go with the preference – it is how your spine wants to behave and will benefit from the freedom and fluidity. The healing power of the waves can be profound; explore the possibilities – it's not yours – but an invitation to observe an ancient creature.

The mechanical aspects of practice present another door. In passing through it, we realise a freer way of being. The central mechanism provides a way out of the habitual self and into the organism. Analysis, whether anatomical or psychological, is divisive, as it disturbs our sense of unity. But each time we practise, analysis gives us a starting point and is the companion of our enquiry. As we proceed, we divide and unite, separate and come together again. As our inner dance moves between polarities, we discover that depth is limitless, vast and timeless.

Your Research

Preamble

> *Personal research forms an experiential basis for all we impart. The inspiration to act and teach is driven by an ever-deepening consequence of our inquiry.*

This quote, from Georg Feuerstein's book *Lucid Waking*, will resonate. He quotes the Bulgarian spiritual teacher Omraam Mikhael Aivanhov:

The artist par excellence is he who takes his own flesh as material for his sculpture, his own face and body as a canvas on which to paint, his own thoughts and feelings as clay to be modelled. He wants all the beauty and harmony of creation to flow and be expressed through his being. An artist such as this creates the art of the new culture which is dawning ... A human being who becomes a living masterpiece, who writes the book of himself, does far more for mankind than all the libraries, museums and works of art in the world, for they are dead and he is alive (Feuerstein 1997).

This could not be closer to the 'fact of practice'. Although the *idea is not the experience* we can start with an *idea* of mechanical, organic and fluid properties. Bony organisation, tissue activity and fluidisation may become part of the language used in our thought feelings and in teaching. The idea becomes the experience. These elements, going back through bone, tissue and fluid — the way we came, from the womb, from the oceans — provide an endless source of practical material. If a 'spiritual dimension arises' the experience is enhanced.

We each have our own practice and style. This section may underpin your own work or be used as a practice on its own merits. The text leading up to and following the practical applications may be of interest to all those involved in body-mind work.

Not everyone practises from a book. It is not possible to convey the subtle elements of sensory experience by the written word. A whole page could be devoted to repeating one or two suggestions. This is what it might take to begin to convey a deeper, more integrated sensory experience. You cannot hold a book and 'go within', but you can read the text, imbibe the idea of the sensations, feel through thought feelings, and then practically explore them. You are invited.

The basic positions follow the fact that all postures and movements arise from the basic attitudes of lying, sitting, all-fours, kneeling, crouching and standing. Depth work is best approached in these positions because they are mechanically easy to use, not challenged by range of movement, and provide access to the central mechanism without the additional distraction of 'how to do a posture'.

Start from *who* you are. Begin with gravitation and breathing and move into the mechanical activity of your bones and the organic quality of your tissues. The positions, attitudes and the possibilities within them present no challenge. Range of movement is secondary. Give up your postures for a while. Undercut a desire to make expansive movements by coming back in to yourself. Begin positional work with an element of containment. Everything that is *done* is intended to reveal original qualities and new possibilities. The slight repositioning of an arm, leg, or spine can shift the focus, go deeper and wake up another element. Positions, breathing and their possibilities bring out a vital activity that underscores the positions. The work is physiological as opposed to physical. At one and the same time we are guests, mentors and students of our bodies. Be completely attentive to the depth of sensory information to maximise organic and mechanical potential; allow your body to draw you in and go to meet it.

This work encourages a proliferation of involuntary movement. Balance voluntary organisation with involuntary responses. Appeal to the innate understanding of the organism. You do not have to do all the suggested positions and variations as a sequence. Try one or two and go deeply for short periods. Each position, angle, suggestion and nuance that arises through self-discovery becomes another framework for sensory awareness to find more subtlety.

Treat every position, change of angle, configuration, and each breath as if they are new experiences – don't know them or it. *The organism speaks from its own place.*

'Intimacy' implies deep understanding. Working intimately takes us to the essential nature of the organism, and the deeper you go the more responsive it becomes. The more deeply we work, the more we stimulate the organism to return its intelligence to our awareness. It keeps coming back to the local and peripheral associates of the diaphragm and spine, which connect and draw on the whole body.

Separate yourself from something more ancient than yourself. Stand back, feel from a distance, and then join a deep articular dance. Your sensory possibilities include skin, myofascial activity, bone and fluidisation. Combine the possibilities with changes in bony position – this cannot be taught – only you know through feeling what the moment-to-moment requirements are; take responsibility for your sensations

You have choices of position, subtle adjustments, rate of breathing and length of respiratory pauses. Variations have variable effects and are beyond technique. The following suggestions (as opposed to instructions) do not refer to the gross aspects of positioning which are obvious from the illustrations. The text is aimed at the possibilities, the smaller positional changes and movements. Sometimes you do not need to do that much. When an approach is intelligent, the body-mind will absorb it readily and remember it. When you 'hit the spot', it resonates for some time afterwards because you have awoken an existing intelligence as opposed to performing a specific shape.

The following attitudes are suggestions. We can invite primal activity from any attitude, exploring a wide range of spontaneous movement as the body and breath find their depth and direction.

The Dynamics of Supination

Lying down is a key position and one we keep returning to between the other positions. It is not resting: in fact, far from it. Supination is used in all body work because it induces relaxation and reduces tension in the postural muscles. Although relaxation is an element, the skeletal framework, articulations and soft tissues are activated by the breath and contact with the ground (See Figures 16.1-4).

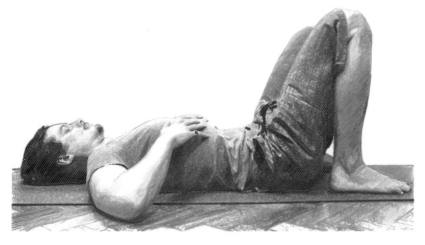

Figure 16.1

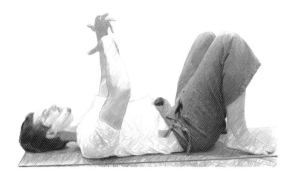

Figure 16.2

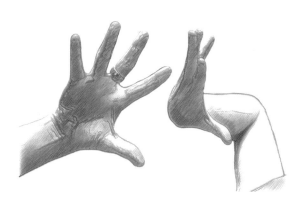

Figure 16.3

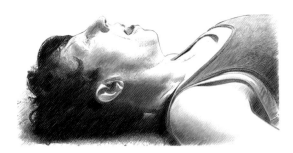

Figure 16.4

Note: The clawed-finger attitude of the fingers on the lower ribs — the proximity of the heels to the pelvis — the slight extension of the neck, like a creature waiting to receive something (an inhalation, a morsel, an impulse from below) — work your feet, lift the arches and create space in the ankles — spread the toes, anchor the base of your big toes to the ground — release your jaw — soften your face and your inner voice — follow the shape of your bones.

The work of the feet and ankles comes up into the pelvis and beyond, into your spine and shoulders. Now go into your thoracic diaphragm — it is stimulated by the deep action of your feet and hands — the connective tissue covering the feet and hands resemble diaphragms and are directly connected to the thoracic and pelvic diaphragms. Go deeply into your exhalation and *wait* — for the deep engagement to take off.

Remember to activate the area around your epiglottis, creating a soft valve for your diaphragm and abdominal tissue to work against. This creates a deeper and stronger action.

Feel the deep engagement of the diaphragm and abdominal muscles while you wait — feel the spread throughout all articulations, the spine, the tissues and your skin. The diaphragm acts as a pump, drawing fluids up through the major vessels, vena cava and lymphatic duct but also acts as a spinal, thoracic and abdominal pump, creating a powerful rhythm throughout the whole of the body's skeletal and soft tissue arrangement. You might play with slow, long pauses for the organism to turn itself around for the inhalation or a more rapid rhythmic action to 'get things moving'.

Yield all your impediments to the ground for your inhalation to come in — pass through distractions with your sensory mind surrendering. It is more natural for the organism to surrender than it is for the mind. The mind holds the organism back.

Physical impediments to a deeper and more naturally expansive breath are confined to the local respiratory areas such as diaphragm, deep hip flexors, abdominal and accessory muscles, and also the spinal muscles but, as the breath spreads, restrictions between any vertebrae from the sacrum to the occiput, upper or lower ribs, shoulder or pelvic girdles and the jaw can be restrictive. As practice deepens, it becomes clearer to what extent the movement of the sacrum at the sacroiliac joints is involved in freedom of the breath.

It begins as the idea of practice, before long you drop the idea and are no longer practicing, but taking part in something more intelligent than you are. The deeper you go the further back in time you go, beyond ideas and beyond practice. As 'a spine' becomes more alive inside you the more you are in tune with an ancient inherency.

You are drawn to the movement of bones, as they settle in gravity, the activity of all tissues between your skin and your spine and back again. When you have engaged with several breaths with long pauses, you could 'play' with your diaphragm before the inhalation arrives: invite it to move a little faster, slow it down again, it's up to you when to move between engagement and a fluid pumping action.

Change the position of your arm (See Figure 16.7) — note the palm is turned upward with only the back of the wrist touching your chest. The heel on the same side is lifted — the front of the foot is deeply engaged with the ground. Slowly draw the heel back and down to open and lift the arch — sustain the deep space you have created in the ankle — the movement comes up through your skin, articulations and bones into your shoulder (and potentially jaw). Keeping the tension in the foot and palm, your arm will slowly unfold as your shoulder blade is drawn into

your spine during the pause. Be attentive to your tail bone — feel its rhythm.

Try some alternative arm positions which change the inner space dynamic (See Figures 16.5 and 6) — the arms unfold from the spine, for the inhalation to arrive — the mechanics of movement obey the needs of the organism for oxygen. *Give your bones away to receive them again — centre your bones.*

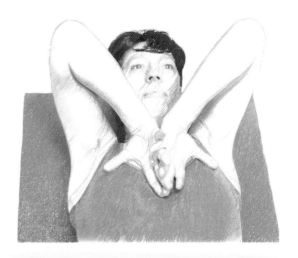

Figure 16.5

Figure 16.6

An Alternative arm and hand attitude.

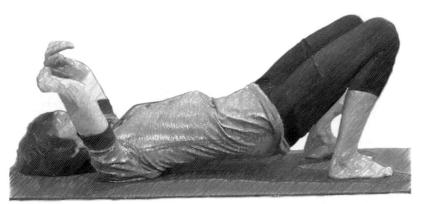

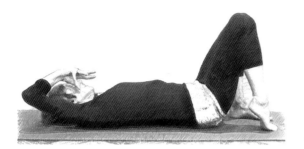

Figure 16.7

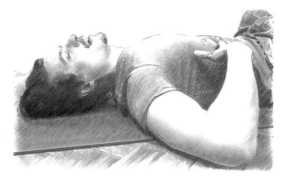

Figure 16.9

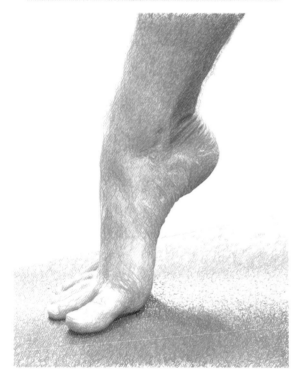

Figure 16.8

A working foot.

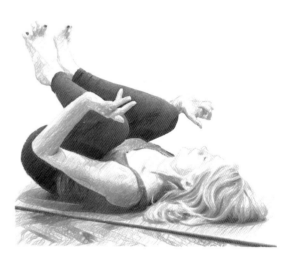

Figure 16.10

Breathe deeply and pleasurably to feel the changes. Tune in to the respiratory movements of your skin and bones, and the activity of your tissues (see Figure 16.9).

Fold completely – be tight like a ball (see Figures 16.10 and 11) – touch the front of the lumbar curve with the exhalations and unfold during the pauses – engaging deeply through the front of your spine.

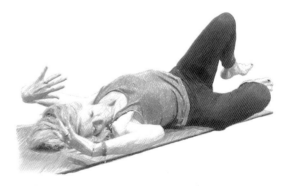

Figure 16.11

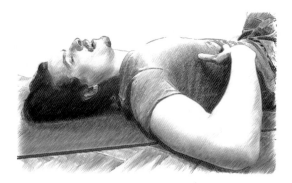

Figure 16.12

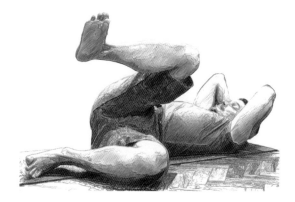

Figure 16.15

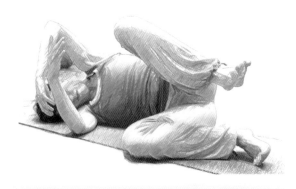

Figure 16.13

Repeating the basic lying attitude (see Figure 16.12) gives an opportunity for re-evaluation and the emergence of insights. Insights are a consequence of positive activity releasing into awareness as we remove and sink beneath habitual patterns — most insights reflect the same meaning.

Working on your Side

Note the position of the under leg and the engagement of the small toe (See Figures 16.13 - 15). Bring

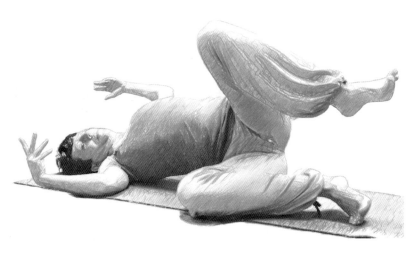

Figure 16.14

Opening from the center.

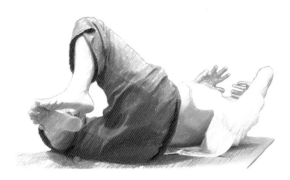

Figure 16. 16

Once we accept that everything is connected by bone, tissue, nerve, fluid and biochemistry, once we acknowledge that we are all connected and interdependent and that we are connected to universal elements because we share universal constituents, we can get on with the business of *feeling it.* Unfold actively from deep action (see Figures 16.16 -17).

Drop all concepts and move on to the next inhalation! Start again, clear the way for an unknown experience. It is more natural for the organism to surrender than for the mind. The mind holds the organism back.

Return to Figure 16.18 and re-evaluate your articular dance, depth of action and inner space.

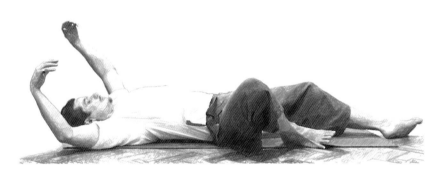

Figure 16.17

Extending from deep action.

the upper leg towards your chin. Keep hands and feet actively open and working. Feel free to rotate your head in a way that brings your neck into the movement from below. Come back to the diaphragm, the abdominal tissue, the pause. *Each exhalation brings tail and head towards each other and each inhalation separates them – this is primal activity – the spine folds and unfolds with the breath - the tail continues to move rhythmically.*

Remember to give your contact points to the ground. 'Contain' your shoulder girdle by keep the elbows close. During the pause, rotate slowly – the tail continues to move with the breath. Rotation is enhanced just before, as the inhalation returns the spine to extension (rotation is augmented by extension as the deep spinal tissues release).

Note the arm and head possibilities – be creative – fold – unfold. The rotation comes by itself – rotation activates, imbibes and nourishes the discs.

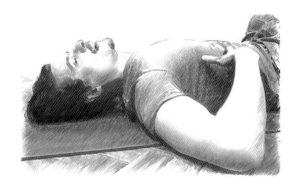

Figure 16.18

The Power of Pronation

Unfolding from pronation can be a powerful movement. It is a primal action (Figures 16.19-21). We are trying to get up, but the abdominal wall potentially weakens if it falls forward and the diaphragm loses its purchase on the spine. The back of the body compensates by overworking, easily compressing the vertebrae.

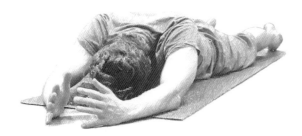

Figure 16.19

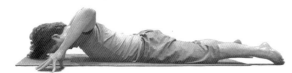

Figure 16.20

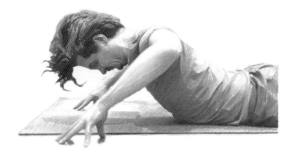

Figure 16.21

The breath is instrumental in moving the tail, sacrum and spine; the upper body lifts 'by itself' for the inhale – a creature reflexively seeking something! Note the variation in arm positions. Hand contact with the ground may use the fingers, the outer edge of the hand or flat of the palm. Each variation alters the orientation of the shoulder girdle in relation to the spine. The shoulders and dorsal spine and head receive from the arms and from all the pelvic articulations — the tissues of the thighs and pelvic floor draw up from active feet. The shoulder blades are key players in action — relax your facial muscles - release your jaw — soften your inner voice! The tail continues to move with the breath — introduce some side bending — the entire back of the body including the inner thigh tissue pulls itself together on the out-breath — your tailbone spontaneously flexes and extends. Move between your bones.

Evolving to All-Fours

This is a simple attitude full of possibilities (Figures 16.22-16.26). Continue to allow the sensations and activity of skin, superficial fascia, overall tissue, deep articular space and spinal sensations to pass through awareness.

Note: bent elbows encourages shoulder release — the outer hand and little finger contact with the ground to free the shoulder blades — keep hands and fingers active — release your neck and jaw — give and receive through your contact points.

Move into the back of your body from the front as you unfold from the anterior spine. Keep bringing the belly back into the back of the waist and upwards towards your deep shoulders. As the back of your waist opens up from the inside, everything opens up with it — feel the separation of your spinal vertebrae.

Your exhalation draws the entire abdominal area, pubis and solar plexus up and back towards the spine, creating a deep 'hump'. The skin tightens on the back of the body as if the spine is trying to break through — hold during the pause and continue to deepen and spread internally through the back of your rib cage. Your tail and head have moved towards each other for an out-breath — and then the tail is proactive as the spine lifts and releases back into extension.

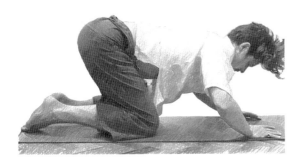

Figure 16.22

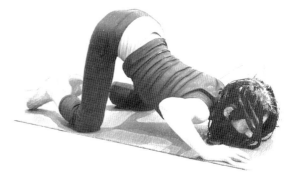

Figure 16.24

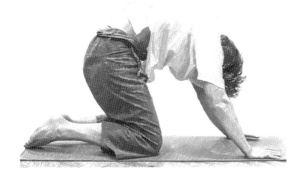

Figure 16.23

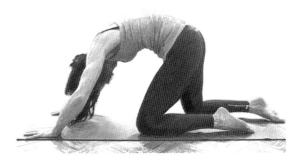

Figure 16.25

Figure 16.26

On all fours and fingertips.

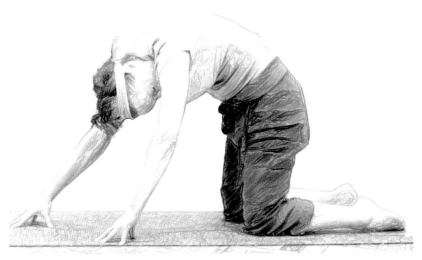

The spine releases into extension for the inhalation – the tail and head move away from each other – once again a primal organic action, the spine is respiratory, and respiration is spinal.

The spinal dynamic is changed by placing the arms, legs and pelvis in a variety of positions – as well as resting in gravity, you are also drawing away from the ground into the spinal vertebrae and dome of the diaphragm.

Let go to the rhythm of the spine – feel every vertebra pick up the action – move rhythmically through your naturally flexible and rigid areas, enabling them to blend in one wave-like movement.

Return to Figure 16.27: re-evaluate texture, articular rhythm, space and the beginning of fluidity – softness arrives.

Wilhelm Reich points out in *Character Analysis* (Reich 1942) 'We already know that the attitude of inhalation is the most important instrument in the suppression of *any* kind of emotion.'

Combining the anatomical map and sensory intelligence enhances awareness. Once you pass beyond a certain point, the map becomes redundant. The entire organism loses its anatomical differentiation as our fluid nature takes over.

Convergence is the key; everything comes together, to the same point, and then opens into space.

Unfolding from the Ground

Evolution unfolded us; it took millions of years to stand up. The spine unfolded by developing anterior curves and moved away from the pelvis with the assistance of the deep respiratory muscles. The entire body unfolded; the action was deep and powerful and took its cue from the ground and from the lumbar spine.

Unfold from the ground very slowly by releasing the knees at their contact points (See Figures 16.28 and 29). Rest on the outer edges of your hands with active fingers. Your heels extend back and down from the base of the big toes – keep your knees bent – draw up through the skin at front of your shins and top of your feet – the arches become deep and strong – the breath will move your spine into flexion and extension and this will be transmitted rhythmically to your knees and elbows – don't stretch your legs but let them work in concert with your lumbar curve – your arms work rhythmically with your dorsal curve.

Connective tissue draws up through the long bones into your shoulders, pelvis and spine. The feet work

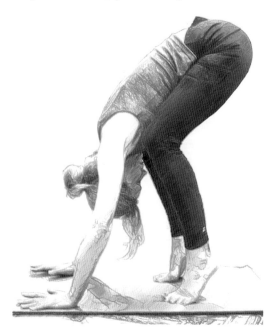

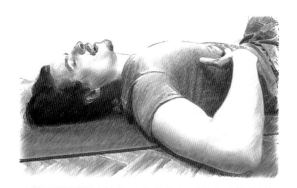

Figure 16.27

Figure 16.28

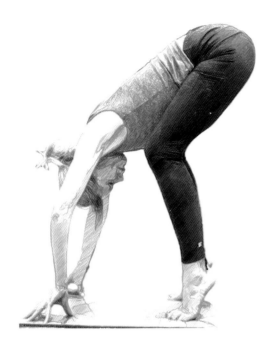

Figure 16.29

tissue and articular relationship that make up the central mechanism for moving and breathing under the earth's pull are found within the deep lumbar and dorsal spine, and they are accessible to awareness. We evolved from enfoldment and proceeded to unfold. Unfolding is an original expression. We can re-establish the power of unfolding before we fold or bend. We can restore the strength and centring needed to move away from the ground.

Don't be fooled by the apparent simplicity of this movement (Figure 16.30), it is mechanically powerful and important, as it engages the entire system upward from the feet, and centrally from the spine towards the ground and the head. The lower body must work to maintain space in the foot and leg articulations.

Note the proximity of the finger tips to the toes — keep the shoulder blades soft and receptive, the knees bent and wider than the feet — release your head, neck and jaw. Work from the centre of your feet to place your heels down from the front of your spine, and go s-l-o—w—l—y. Your diaphragm and abdominal muscles 'draw up' the tissue wrapped around your entire legs and the dorsum of the foot — into, through and around your pelvis. *Engage the depth body while waiting for the inhale.* Keep your weight slightly forward to enable the base of the big toe to engage with your diaphragm.

hard at first — activating the arch, the toes, and creating deep space in the ankles. What begins as a voluntary position becomes an involuntary event involving the spine and breath. You are working with superficial tissue, myofascial activity and articular space and rhythm — the long bones give to, and receive from, the spine. *Stop thinking — become a creature — allow thoughts to be feeling thoughts without language.*

Breathe deeply and voluminously to feel the changes to space and softness. Follow the pause easily and freely and just allow it. You will recognise the point where it needs to leave you as it sinks quietly into the unknown depths of your physiology. *The elements of deep pausing can only be, and should remain, unknown.* Focus on the *texture* of your sensations as they radiate from an intelligence within and spread from a deep fluid base to your skin. Go with the deeper rhythms arising from your spine, allowing your arms to move in concert with your breath — be a creature.

The physiological elements most immediately accessible and potentially responsive to the needs of the organism are those involved in movement on land, notably gravitation and breathing. The bones, reflexive

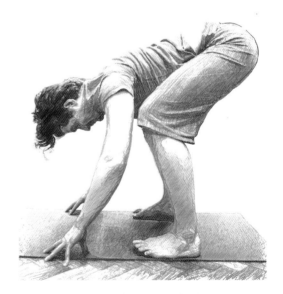

Figure 16.30

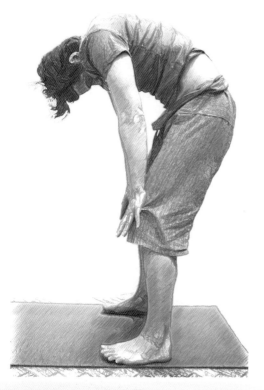

Figure 16.31

As you unfold and *the entire spine moves inward* from the tail and sacrum, there is the possibility of moving into more extension — stay strong and deep — the pause is essential as it reinforces the spine through the diaphragm and abdominal muscles. Release for the inhalations and re-engage on the exhalations. You may choose to rhythmically integrate the entire body, arches to jaw by pumping the diaphragm and abdominals — you will come up spontaneously (see Figures 16.31-16.34). If the control is there you may find yourself moving into an extension beyond the normal upright posture — but don't bend backwards — as it disconnects your body from your axis — the action is at the front of you body — and the knees, which must support you, function from the feet and the central activity of the spine and the breath. Note the slight flexion of the hips and knees in order to maximise the engagement of the central mechanism. You are effectively moving towards reversing your spinal curves. This demands a strong purchase from the feet and legs. We unfolded from the earth.

If you try to forward bend from this position, keeping your knees slightly bent, you will feel the articulatory depth and space as you fold.

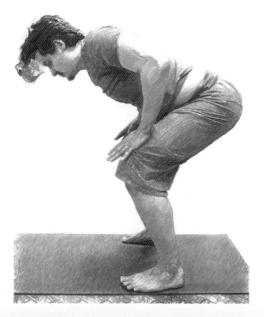

Figure 16.32

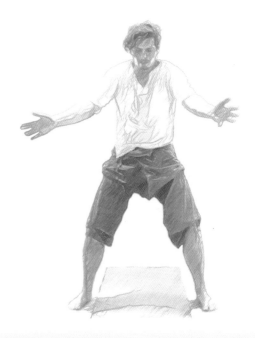

Figure 16.33

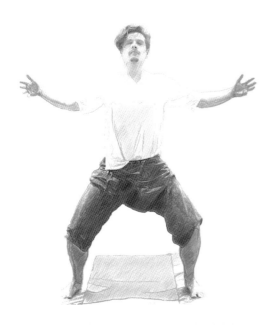

Figure 16.34

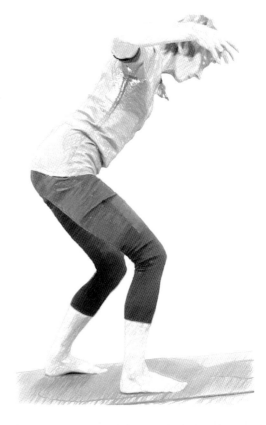

Figure 16.36

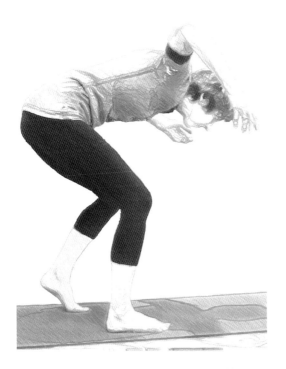

Figure 16.35

Unfold while focusing more on one leg, i.e. the right leg, drawing up through the long tissue of the thigh from an active foot and ankle. You will spontaneously rotate to the right. This is a primal action – the spine rotates and the shoulders open in response to the exaggerated action of the right leg.

Unfolding with one leg forward invites the same mechanism (Figures 16.35–37). Note the heel position – remember to keep the feet and toes open to begin with – lift the arches without lifting the toes. There is substantial potential for expansion in the upper body coming up through the articular space, and tissue engagement. See how it feels when you alternate enhancing the action on each leg. The spine will turn either way – and the arms will open spontaneously from the sacrum and spine.

Come back to Figure 16.38, and breathing voluminously and purposefully; feel the softening and space from

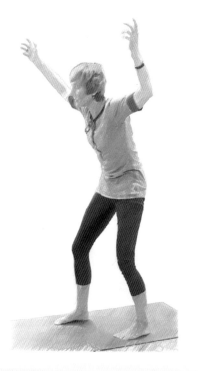

Figure 16.37

Weak and Strong Sides (Everyone has a Scoliosis)

Unfold again with legs slightly further apart and feet slightly turned out (like a dancer) – unfold primarily from one leg and then the other (Figures 16.39–42). Which is your weaker side? The arch, ankle, leg, pelvis and spine will always be weaker on one side, consequently reducing the potential space throughout that side – usually up into the jaw. Everyone has a scoliosis, albeit mild in some, but nevertheless existent. Work on the weak side from the ground up and from the diaphragm and abdominal tissues. The central mechanism on the weak side is invited to work. *As you open powerfully from your centre on the more operative side, the foot is planted into the ground.*

Lie down again as in Figure 16.43.

Use some variations and voluminous pleasurable breaths to consolidate the work – and then calm it down to involuntary expression.

The mind, with its positive and negative aspects, has unfolded as a consequence of gravitation and respiration. Physiology is *more* powerful than the thinking, feeling mind because it has, among other things, the

within and the aliveness of your spine – *don't know it* – as the involuntary movements take off. Calm it down, gravitate, feel the bones, articulations and fluid move inside you and your skin receive the deeper activity.

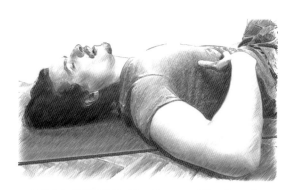

Figure 16.38

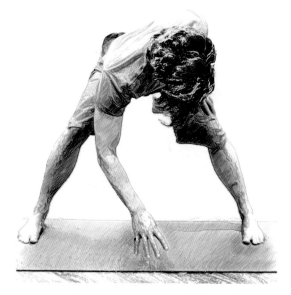

Figure 16.39

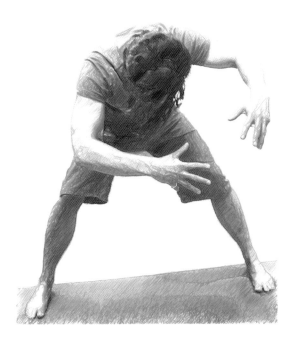

Figure 16.40

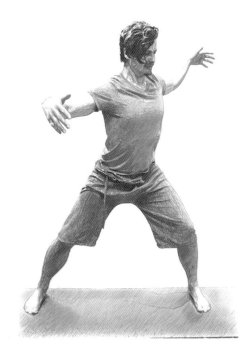

Figure 16.42

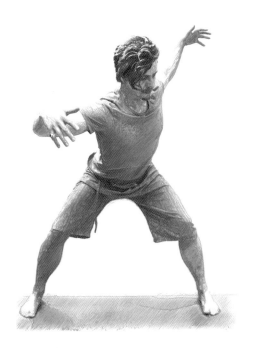

Figure 16.41

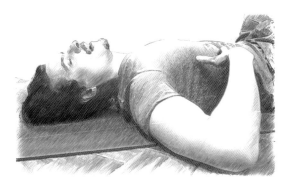

Figure 16.43

additional property of 'innocence'. We can revert to innocence by immersing ourselves in physiology. Innocence simply registers sensation without comparison or analysis. Innocence wonders at deep fluid activity.

Tissue drawing bone – skin drawing tissue – bones dance with breath – deep articular engagement and space – total sensory predominance – the witness leaves – you are a creature!

Generally, we see and feel what we are conditioned to see and feel. When we look beneath our initial impressions and sink below expected sensations, we make space for the emergence of insight and understanding to emerge — step aside, and then step aside from stepping aside. Original activity has not been modified by experience, learning or knowledge; it is instinctive. We have grown up out of the ground and from surrounding space.

In life we have a tendency towards collapse. We hold ourselves up with the outer body/tissues while unknowingly allowing the deeper tissues to weaken. This can occur on both sides, but to a larger extent it often occurs on only one side. By this point in your practice, your sensations may have deepened, with a softer, more complete integration from the soles of the feet up through the pelvic and thoracic diaphragms into the dorsal spine and shoulders. This again is an essential movement, as it recapitulates our evolution to the upright position.

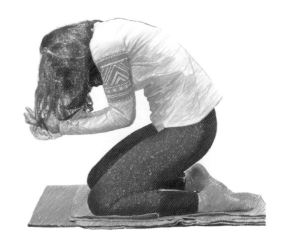

Figure 16.44

On the Knees

This strong position needs work. Unfold from almost all fours (Figures 16.44-46) — the abdominal muscles work with the diaphragm to *inhibit bending backwards* — your tail and head move towards each other on the exhale — the spine moves in to follow the tail and sacrum as the diaphragm lifts and spreads its wings — the tail and sacrum move inwards — the entire central mechanism sucks back and up from the solar plexus, navel and lower belly to support and open the vertebrae. This is a deep and contained unfoldment; note the slight flexion of the hips to engage the central mechanism more fully.

The working relationship between surface and deep tissue, articular space, the ground and the breath is particularly relevant in this attitude.

Be inside your pelvis. You can feel the sacroiliac joints working. Go with the strong myofascial gathering up through the thighs. The pelvic floor is strong and active and the abdominal tissues have their work to do — once you have engaged you can release for the inhale and re-engage for the exhale. You can only do

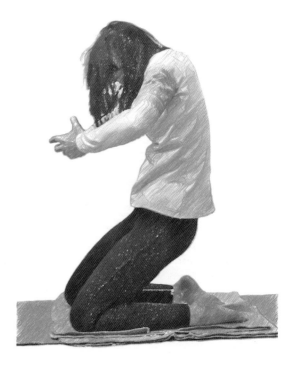

Figure 16.45

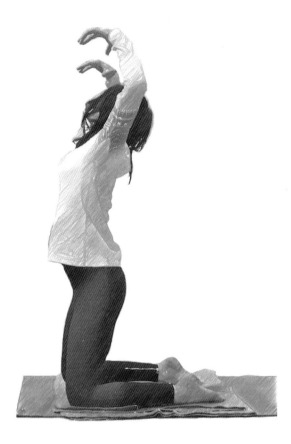

Figure 16.46

formation – and even more relevant – the process of unrolling, opening out, disengaging from an envelope. In geometry evolution means 'the unfolding of a curve'. Evolve means to disentangle, to bring out (what exists implicitly and potentially). These terms can be used to describe body-mind experiences that arise during practice. In practice, we evolve in reverse – we shed the tensions resulting from our conditioning and return to a less impaired state, to more of an original condition – we restore ourselves.

When the spine dances to its own tune, we do not need to add that many postures, and may not need to practise for that long. Active freedom in its original state has revealed itself. Does a snake move when it has no reflexive need; does it move simply because it can? Does it move spontaneously as an expression of organic pleasure arising from movement itself? Our internal snake has the possibility of such a transformational experience.

Figures 16.48 and 49 appear to be the preparation for a backbend from the ground up. It is, but it is also a working position in itself, without coming up.

Note: the proximity of the feet to the pelvis, the working foot and ankle. The front of the shin is active – your pelvis picks up from your long bones and from the myofascial draw coming up from your arches.

The sacrum and shoulder blades work together – the entire body gathers itself together. Note slight hip flexion to engage the central mechanism. The tail bone moves rhythmically in flexion and extension with the breath, opening and closing the entire spine above.

this once you have adequate support at the front of the body. Don't bend backwards and weaken your axis, but let it come by itself, if at all – the tail and head move towards each other on the out-breaths. Unfolding to an upright position can be adequate when you move from your centre.

Come back to lying down (Figure 16.47). Now, really go deeply with your exhale. Play with the diaphragm – pause for long periods or not at all – bathe in fluidity, which may be profuse. Sensation arose through movement and movement was stimulated by sensation; consciousness arose through both.

Practice is an evolving process and may have some parallels with the evolutionary process itself. Evolution can mean advancement, growth, progression, trans-

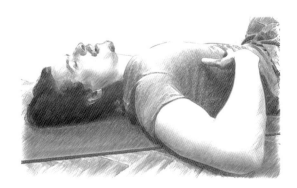

Figure 16.47

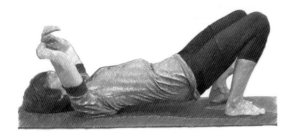

Figure 16.48

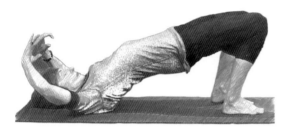

Figure 16.49

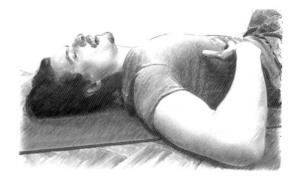

Figure 16.50

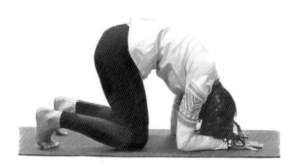

Figure 16.51

Fluidity becomes more prolific – the spine floats. Try a one-sided action: work one wrist, arm, shoulder foot and leg on one side – pull yourself together on one side – your pelvis and shoulder will lift on that side, and you will rotate towards the other side. You can alternate one side to the next, engaging and disengaging in spiral rotations.

Contain yourself. Start small – come into your spine continually – pause for the diaphragm to work. The central mechanism behaves in the same way in all attitudes, but in this case it does so on one side – *the diaphragm and pelvic floor work on one side.*

Go through some more deep exploratory activity (Figure 16.50).

This movement unfolds from the wrists, forearms and elbows (Figure 16.51-3). Note: the work of the feet and ankles – the proximity of the knees and elbows – palms face up, or on the outer edge of your hands. It comes from the solar plexus – the tail move towards the throat on the exhale. This is a working position – if you practice inversions – you might come up from the front of the spine. This section is not intended to 'get you up'; it is another working position – feel your long

bones feeding back through their girdles into the spine – be contained. The knees lift by themselves from an active spine; the forearms are grounded by the breath and from the spine.

Re-evaluate (Figure 16.54) the involuntary mechanism is described by those who work with it as: the brain, intracranial membranes, cerebrospinal fluid, articular mobility of the cranial bones, spinal cord, intraspinal membranes, cerebrospinal fluid, and the articular mobility of the sacrum between the ilia. In other words, and simplified, all the soft tissue of the central nervous system: the fluid that bathes it, membranes that divide it, the bones that house and protect it, and the articulations enabling expansion and movement of the mechanism as a whole. Our attention and immersion are sufficient to enhance the rhythm of the involuntary (primary respiratory) mechanism as it spreads out towards the surface of the body, representing as it does a physiological expression of an original self. We

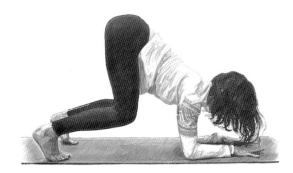

Figure 16.52

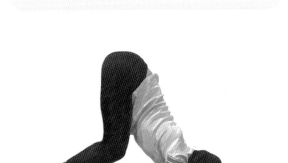

Figure 16.53

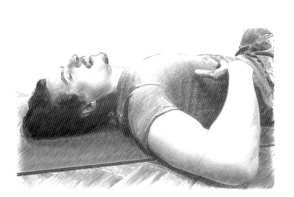

Figure 16.54

can feel our fluid origin pulsate and fluctuate. Involuntary fluid activity provides an ideal focus for non-interference and deep action without doing.

Sit naturally with legs extended (Figures 16.55 and 56).

Note: The turn-out of the thighs — the bend in the knees — the half-point of the feet, like a dancer with toe separation — the action between the large and lesser toes connects to the diaphragm — the breath moves you — tail to head and away again. Your spine moves inwards and upwards for an in-breath — the whole spine from tail to skull moves rhythmically in an undulating wave as you fold and open, and fold again from your solar plexus. Explore arm variations to avoid stagnation.

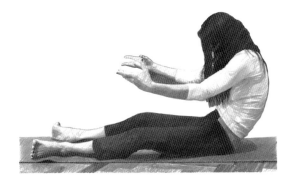

Figure 16.55

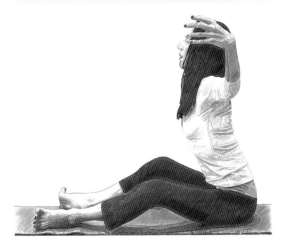

Figure 16.56

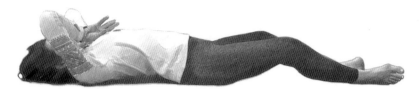

Figure 16.57

Patterning tends to occur in the voluntary muscles, the muscles that we can use to inhibit unwanted sensations or portray the kind of persona we think necessary to give an impression of how we are. The voluntary control acts from the surface and contains the impulse to act that comes from within (Lowen 1958).

Lie down, legs turned out, (see Figure 16.57) maintain the action of the hands and feet — work your diaphragm and abdominal muscles in order to move the entire internal body. Without a mat, and given a smooth floor, the body will move across the floor by itself as the spine rediscovers its reptilian nature. Return to Figure 16.58.

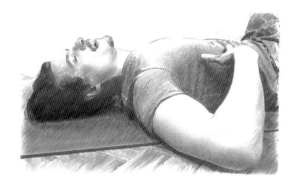

Figure 16.58

Primordial peace, a stillness and healing, arise from involuntary movement. The calmer we are, the greater we can detect the amplitude of involuntary movement. The more prolific the movement, the calmer and more still we become. Physiological stillness is contained within the tides of fluid expression.

Releasing tension releases something in the tissues, an endorphin perhaps, that could be called the chemical of wisdom. As physical tone and texture soften and open, insights find space, arising in consciousness as if the soul or spirit resides in the cells, and in the fluid that bathes them.

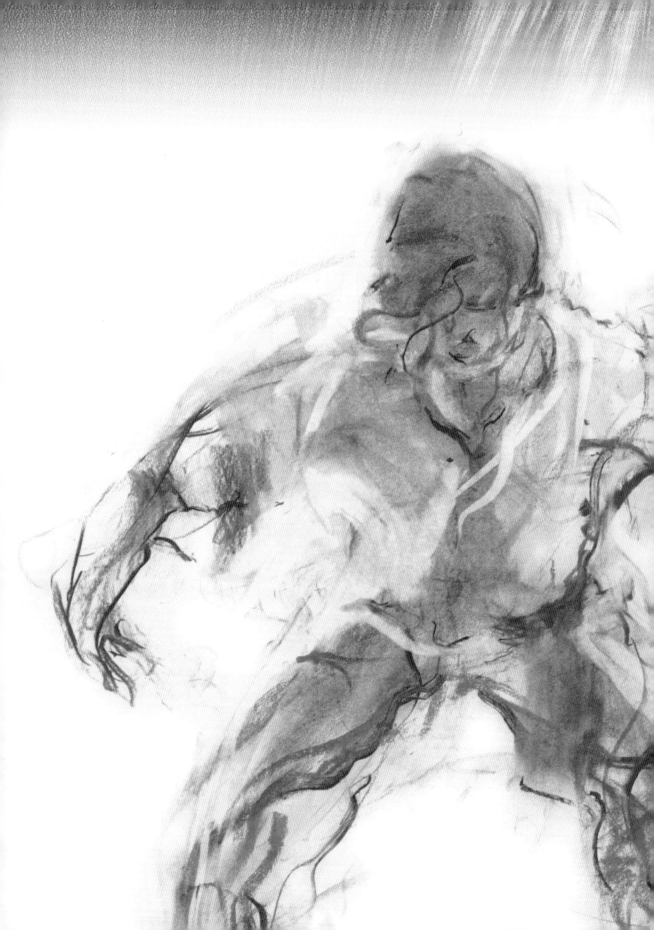

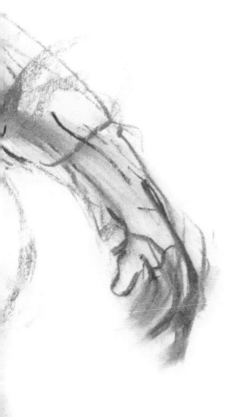

What Lies Beneath?

Suitable Candidates

What lies beneath, an altered state, an alternative consciousness, a variation in behaviour, more love?

Growing up in a tiny apartment with a Jewish mother and grandmother made me a perfect candidate for yoga. No father present or sighted, and bordering on poverty, things could have been worse. Childhood included boils, warts, chronic bronchitis, allergies, depression and a lack of confidence. There has been work to do!

In 1974, with a damaged lumbar disc and a penchant for introspection, I met Lolly, my wife, who introduced me to yoga. She was part of a group of yoga teachers, psychotherapists and writers with R.D. Laing as the central figure. It felt like coming home. The combination of the physiological awakening provided by yoga, and the deep interest in 'how we are' inspired by Laing (Ronnie) was transformational. I willingly did the work. More than 40 years later I am still doing it, but from another place, a place that has generated this book.

Regardless of personal history, we are all suitable candidates for change. If you are reading this, you are working with the physical aspect, have an interest in the philosophy and are aware of permutations on other levels. The fundamental principle holds true: 'you can only find it in and for yourself'. We keep coming back to us, returning to our own experience.

Changing the body changes how we are. At first the changes can be extraordinary. The centring, ground-ing, release of tension and sensitivity touches all levels. As time goes by we grow used to the changes. Old patterns, recurrent and stirred by circumstance, may be well established.

We approach our body and self with authenticity and a penetrating interest. We may know intuitively what lies beneath the skin. If change is not anticipated or considered necessary, it may occur of its own accord. Deeper work addresses the grip of the past.

Self-Interest

It begins and ends with our self. A self is defined as 'one's own person' or as 'an individual as the object of his or her own reflective consciousness'. *Having a self implies there is a part of oneself that is the owner of the self that one has.* There is more to us than ourself.

Yogis were self-interested, proposing that the self is illusory and open to transcendence. An ambitious project, this self doesn't feel illusory, but may benefit from some refinement. In reality we are never free from self-interest because the process of yoga demands the practice of passing through our ever-present self. All experience is self-experience. We are always 'there'; even when we are 'out of our heads' a part of us records the experience.

Selves arise out of living tissue; working with tissue has a direct and accumulative effect on the self. This is obvious through personal experience and a well-established fact in the body-mind world. As body work does its job, the neocortex loosens its grip. Changes to behaviour, temperament and understanding are par for the course.

An original self is not free from cortical presence, but has a mature relationship with it. We draw from subcortical activity, learning from ancient rhythms untouched by agendas. The older and the more recent aspects are intimately connected, inseparable, and belong to the same organic fabric. The brain, from bottom up, is a continuum.

Wiping the Slate

Wiping the physiological slate clean gives a sense of freedom from ourselves *at the time*. Can an original self arise out of an original body? Deeper patterns dissolve in the wake of original physical experience but we must be present to have the experience. A less conditioned way of being needs recognition if it is to be adopted.

When we 'surrender' to the body and give over to primal movement, *when we have gone*, a familiar self springs back, as if on a piece of elastic. We are an ever-present polarity between our habitual and original self. Time spent has an accumulative effect and we do recognise the changes.

We are not just organisms. R.D. Laing writes, in his classic *The Divided Self*:

One's relationship to an organism is different to one's relationship to a person ... One acts towards an organism differently from the way one acts towards a person. The science of persons is the study of human beings that begins from a relationship with the other person and proceeds to an account of the other still as a person. 'In man seen as an organism therefore, there is no place for his desires, fears, hope or despair as such' (Laing 1960).

Laing points out the necessity for us to see ourselves as we are. Negation is not the answer, while acceptance of our frailty might be the place to start.

Laing was a master at listening to vulnerable people. We might be, or might become, more masterful at listening to what goes on within and between us. This demands respect and sensitivity. Yoga draws attention to, and aims in part to, potentially dissolve the complex-ity, ambiguity and confusion arising out of our desires, fears, hopes and despairs. We can move towards this by perceiving ourselves as organisms but with a sensitivity, presence and underlying innocence. (Laing spent time in India and saw the benefits in yoga practice. During their time in therapy with him, he would often recommend his clients to a yoga teacher.) We can return to a former state and dissolve conditioning (to the extent that this is possible), reinforce ourselves with organic power, and start again.

Wilhelm Reich and Alexander Lowen employed the 'organism approach'. Lowen writes: 'In pose, in posture, in attitude and in every gesture, the organism speaks a language which antedates and transcends its verbal expression' (Lowen 1958). Reich, like Laing and many others, was influenced by Freud but saw a need to work with the body in tandem with psychoemotional work. Reich writes:

We no longer work merely on individual conflicts and special armourings but on the living organism itself ... The idea of orthodox psychology and depth psychology are chained to word formations. However the living organism functions beyond all verbal ideas and concepts. Human speech, a biological form of expression at an advanced stage of development, is not a specific attribute to the living organism, which functions long before a language and verbal representations exist. ... many animals express themselves through sounds, but the living organism functioned prior to and functions beyond the use of sounds as a form of expression (Reich 1942).

Reich saw that authentic organic expression could be blocked by patterns of tension. He continues:

The beginning of living function lies much deeper than and beyond language. Over and above this, the living organism has its own modes of expressing movement which simply cannot be comprehended with words. ... human language also often functions as a defence. The spoken word conceals the expressive language of the biological core (Reich 1942).

Reich used verbalisation in his therapeutic approach but not until the armour attached to the emotional block had been loosened. In our case, loosening of the deeper recesses of our organic nature may be sufficient in addressing aspects of personal history. If and when psychotherapy is in progress, the physical changes provide a helpful adjunct to treatment by loosening the defensive tensions that support psychoemotional patterns. Reich saw a need for restoring motility to the plasma of the body and sought to bring out the full pulsatile quality of his patient's physiology.

Originally there was no self. The organism is original. The intention is not to lose consciousness, but to drop habitual thought in order to absorb the unconditioned freedom of spontaneous movement. If we start with the premise that the organism is benevolent, we can enter into it as it presents itself. We may underestimate the properties of the organism with regard to it having a self. Is there an organic self that lies dormant regardless of practice and sometimes in spite of it?

One Consciousness

We experience consciousness and consciousness enables experience. The fields of consciousness and experience are the same. We may not experience the physiology of consciousness but feel conscious. The quality of consciousness may vary. Yoga suggests that we are not fully conscious, that we are in a sleeping state. A sense of awakening is the common experience.

We can feel the depth and quality of another person's consciousness. Consciousness has a quality that may be felt in others. The more consciously aware someone is the more we feel it. We feel it in people from all walks of life, and it is particularly noticeable in charismatic individuals and spiritual teachers. Consciousness can shine or not.

R.D. Laing recounts meeting Gregory Bateson for the first time as they took an elevator together. Laing describes an atmosphere of silent attentiveness as each assessed the quality of the others consciousness. The intensity of a spiritual teacher's consciousness may reduce his audience to tears before he has spoken. The possibility of sharing collective consciousness led the yogis towards their belief that consciousness existed before the material body. It may feel this way during our more sensitive and awakened moments.

The simplicity of consciousness has been divided into a subconscious, unconscious, pre-conscious, ego-consciousness and super-consciousness, and there may be more. Consciousness may also be personal, collective or universal. Authorities on consciousness, e.g. Freud and Damasio, divide it into layers and tell us that our experience of consciousness arises from upper, more recent layers of a nervous system built upon a hierarchy of lower, more ancient layers of which we have, limited, if any, experience. While philosophers, scientists, yogis and psychoanalysts deliberate over the nature of consciousness, we understand consciousness through direct experience. Experience does not explain consciousness; it is consciousness. One possible definition of consciousness is 'an organism's awareness of its own self and surroundings'. Based on our own experience and with respect to anatomical and functional divisions within the nervous system, *there is one consciousness*, although we may not be aware of its entire content. Freud and Patanjali (the father of organised yoga and well known in this field) in their own way, in their own era, compartmentalised consciousness but also recognised that there is one consciousness. Freud compartmentalised consciousness for psychoanalytical purposes, but also recognised it as a continuum, the unconscious, less conscious and fully conscious being part of the same whole (Freud 1927).

Jean Gebser writes: 'There is no so-called unconscious; there are only modalities (or intensities) of consciousness ... Consciousness is not identical with the process of thinking , nor is it limited to the awareness of the ego' (Gebser 1945). His observations could not be more in tune with the Eastern understanding.

Krishnamurti saw an undivided consciousness within each of us. He writes:

Consciousness is the total field in which thought functions and relationships exist, but we have come to divide this consciousness into the active and the dormant, the upper and lower levels – that is all the daily thoughts feelings and activities on the surface and below them the so-called subconscious, the things with which we are not familiar, which express themselves occasionally through certain intimations, intuitions and dreams. ... We have accepted that there is such a thing (as the subconscious) and all the phrases and jargon of the analysts have seeped into the language; but is there such a thing? And why is it that we give such extraordinary importance to it (Krishnamurti 1969).

Krishnamurti writes: 'When you are being totally aware of the whole field of consciousness there is no friction. It is only when you divide consciousness, which is *all* thought, feeling and action, into different levels that there is friction (Krishnamurti 1969). Freud, Krishnamurti, Patanjali and Reich dealt with the human dilemma in different ways, but all felt it necessary to go inwards.

Alexander Lowen cites Erich Newman, author of *The Origins and History of Consciousness*: Consciousness has a twofold aspect. There is first the consciousness of feelings and actions and secondarily, the consciousness of knowing. Newman (Lowen 1958) says: 'The important thing is that consciousness as the acting centre precedes consciousness as the cognitive centre. As this higher ego consciousness develops, it tends to set itself up in opposition to the body, which becomes the representative of the unconscious.'

a stream of consciousness arising from below. Practice opens the ego and enables deeper entry into the body. We pass through the ego to access the deep body and the roots of consciousness that arise from it. It is productive to focus on the skin. As it softens, we also soften the grip of the ego.

Alexander Lowen writes:

The ego must open up its barriers to allow experience in just as it must lower them to allow impulses out. The bigger the experience, the greater the experience must be. This is not a question of flexibility or adaptability, for these involve no change. Literally, an ego must allow itself to be overwhelmed by each new vital experience so that a new ego will arise in which that experience is properly integrated. But this is only possible when the ego extends in depth (Lowen 1958).

Ego Consciousness and the Body

The word *ego* translates from the Latin as 'I myself' and is said to represent the organised part of our personality structure. Ego gives a sense of self, organises our thoughts and is a more recent evolutionary development. The ego is a permanent and necessary fixture, releasing its grip and then returning. It waits in the wings, a tool to be picked up when needed. The ego is the gateway to a deeper expression.

The ego as an upper layer of consciousness was proposed by Freud who also saw it as a body ego (Freud 1927). He writes: 'The ego is ultimately derived from bodily sensations, chiefly those springing from the surface of the body. It may thus be regarded as a mental projection of the surface of the body, besides as we have seen above, representing the superficies of the mental apparatus' (Freud 1927). Freud's observation reminds us that the skin is a derivative of, and unfoldment from, the primary germ layer of tissue the *ectoderm* which produces our central nervous system.

As we *go in* to the body the first thing we meet is the ego, which is stimulated by physical sensation. Ideas, expectations and mental constructs on how to practise come to the forefront of awareness. As we go inwards, it becomes clearer how much of consciousness is taken up by the ego. Ego consciousness is a continuation of

Higher Consciousness

So-called higher consciousness comes from below. Heaven may be above, but above comes from below. The upper layers admit below-ness to conscious awareness. Yoga practitioners have understood that consciousness flows upwards from primal centres long before science examined the nervous system. We loosen the cortical lid to enable the energy to arise from the lower tissues into consciousness. 'Use the body as an instrument of recognition – an instrument to purge the egoistic intelligence' (Iyengar 1987).

'Expanded consciousness' is an emptying of activity. When its content is reduced, consciousness returns to an undisturbed clarity which can be described as intensification. Intensification is not an acceleration of tension but the opposite. We may be reverting to the consciousness of a creature whose senses are undisturbed by cortical activity.

Krishnamurti maintained that all experience is *within* the field of consciousness. In other words, consciousness is not only larger than its content but larger than the experience of itself, an elusive experience of no experience.

Antonio Damasio suggests two forms of consciousness. The consciousness relating to one moment, now, and one place, here, he calls *core consciousness*, which contains no sense of past or future. The other he refers to as *extended consciousness*, which provides the organism with an elaborate sense of self, an identity, a person or a known self. He suggests that core consciousness provides the foundation for extended consciousness. The part of the mind we call self was, biologically speaking, grounded on a collection of non-conscious neural patterns standing for the part of the organism we call the body proper (Damasio 1999).

The consensus is that the unconscious is a filing system (Freud's pre-conscious), some files of experience being less amenable for recall than others, and that there is no unconscious. The entire spectrum of consciousness is like a pond, the murky depths of which are a part of the totality of experience although less accessible. There is, in effect, an unconscious consciousness, containing the history/past experience of the individual and the species. Consciousness is continually reflecting the past as it passes through the present as an unfoldment into the future. Consciousness is a movement.

Sensory Consciousness

In the 1970s, people were experimenting with consciousness by combining yoga practices with LSD. R.D. Laing was using it in controlled therapy sessions. Timothy Leary and Ram Dass were advocating LSD to shift consciousness. For those who experimented, the first casualty of LSD was the ego. Conditioning dissolves as the activity of older centres come to the forefront of awareness; the path is cleared. The senses enliven and take over. Colour, sound, tissue sensations, movements and breathing become intensely magnified. There is an account of a spiritual teacher taking LSD with no effect. In such a case the ego has already been absorbed; consciousness is larger than its content, there is nothing to lose, nothing to break down, and emptiness rules.

I tried LSD once and I felt like warm fluid blending with the space around me. These were the old stretching days. There was no resistance as pure realisation emerged through a melting screen of tension. I became radiant energy. I wrote: 'You just have to be'. This is patently obvious; one *is being* a human being. Two days later, with stiff muscles and a consciousness dulled by extreme exposure, 'just having to be' had lost

its simplicity. It was an interesting experience (not recommended) that had exaggerated an existing awareness that a deep release of tissue tension has a parallel effect on consciousness. Body consciousness is mind consciousness. Something beneath can surface and break the ice.

We can refine consciousness by attending to the body. Consciousness can be perceived as a non-material phenomenon that has arisen from an organic material base. The non-material aspect of consciousness can be approached directly through the material base that generates and sustains it. Consciousness needs living tissue to house it, and from which it can operate and thrive within a strong and vibrant organism. It is well known (to yogis and the like) that energy moving up the spine, culminates in an 'explosion' of consciousness. Damasio writes: 'one of the powerful correlations uncovered so far between brain structure and state of consciousness relates closely to the design for the entry of body signals into the central nervous system' (Damasio 1999). His statement gives credence to the experience of spinal segmentation and the ascendance of sensory nervous activity towards the brain.

Gebser writes: 'Primitive instincts and sublimated processes of thought are simultaneously manifested in the tempero-spatial structure of the central nervous system' (Gebser 1985).

The foundations for conscious awareness are built on an ancient consciousness. We may not have survived the evolutionary mire without being 'unconsciously conscious' of sensations provoked by our environment, i.e. the organisms ongoing responses to external stimuli and an increasing sensitivity to its own sensations. Basic sensory activity is a form of consciousness. Generations of sensory experience have produced consciousness. Antonio Damasio writes: 'Consciousness does depend most critically on regions that are evolutionarily older than more recent, and are located in the depth of the brain rather than its surface' (Damasio 1999). In other words, midline upward extensions of the spinal cord are the forerunners for the development of consciousness.

On the other hand, the yogis may be correct. Perhaps consciousness began as a non-material state. The organism evolved from an energy pattern of consciousness within a grand energy pattern of consciousness. Western consensus disagrees. 'Consciousness has evolved from a non-conscious state' (Damasio 1999).

Consciousness thrives on experience. Consciousness and experience drive each other. Consciousness is a sense that receives information from other senses. An evolving consciousness must have relied on sensory stimulation for its development. Scientific inquiry proposes that the evolutionary basis for consciousness began where incoming sensation became outgoing reaction (Tortora & Anagnostakos 1990). It follows that the augmentation of this meeting place through sensory refinement forms a basis for refining consciousness.

It may not be apparent *when* the roots of consciousness manifested, but it is clearer *where* they sprung from. Antonio Damasio points out that: 'The brain sites associated with core consciousness are located near the brain mid-line. The left and right sides of these structures are like mirror images, looking at each other across the midline. ... These structures are old evolutionary vintage, they are present in numerous non-human species, and they mature early on in individual human development' (Damasio 1999).

The body generates consciousness as a stream of activity coming from a sense of self based on a flow of sensory input. Consciousness arises from organic activity stimulated by our inner and outer environment; consciousness *is* organic activity. 'Consciousness occurs everywhere in our body, not just in our brains. Consciousness at its most basic is 'coherent light' (McTaggart 2001).

Range of consciousness is influenced by the quality of self-awareness, coupled with a sensitivity of the totality of life. Our range of consciousness is influenced by its texture. Consciousness can be sharp, hard, soft or flowing. When the body has soft and deep feelings, consciousness follows suit. A soft and deeply awakened body spreads its conscious energy, touching and being touched by those within its field.

Consciousness is involuntary. We don't *do* consciousness, but we can voluntarily listen to its presence. We can tune in to consciousness to enhance it. Emptying consciousness into the body dissolves conditioning. Primal activity wells up, melting the ego in its wake. Entering the spine awakens consciousness from within by stimulating ancient structures. This forms the basis for light bulb moments in the short term and the potential for deep change in the longer term. People have been pointing this out for centuries.

Physical density inhibits range of consciousness by restricting energetic flow from the body to the brain. Moving deeply uncovers a vital property that renews the system and activates an intelligence that addresses habit. Depth consciousness emerges on waves of pulsations that are free from cortical interference.

The body is organic reality and an ideal source of realisation. The body is now, and its immediacy is the ideal channel for the *sensation of realisation*. 'The implications of life demand that there be no separation between the organism and the psyche. It is a total movement' (Krishnamurti 1969). The body not only gives us an immediate and tangible point of entry; it is the material manifestation of the same energy that generates consciousness.

'What we refer to as mind and consciousness may encompass the totality of communication and regulation in the body, the electromagnetic signatures of countless molecules and atoms and the energy fields they entail' (Oschman 2000).

How Wise is Consciousness?

I would like there to be a consciousness akin to Freud's 'Id' or Damasio's 'core consciousness', but with a sentience, a wisdom, a benevolence. I would like there to be a something within that understands us in spite of ourselves. In practice the body can feel so sensitively responsive that it *feels as if it has its own consciousness*. Krishnamurti, on the *unknown*, writes: 'It is clear that a large part of us is actively awake but beneath a level of consciousness' (1969). To what extent is this wakefulness body consciousness?

Is there a core consciousness that is associated with core power, core fluidity, core aliveness? If so, does this consciousness, once freed, and arising from the depth body, cut through our conditioned consciousness from within? Is there a self-conscious organism that finds it expedient to remain beneath our awareness? Is the body conscious of us being conscious of it?

How wise *is* the wisdom of the body? Is it wise enough to reveal itself only when conditions are favourable? Is the organism aware of the invasive nature of the neo-cortex and its need for analysis? Has the body found it necessary to protect itself against the invasive tendencies of its guest, the cortical self? Is the organism a self in its own right conscious of its existence?

The organism survived its environment for millennia before the advent of the cortex; perhaps, among other things, it is now in the process of surviving it. Should we preserve the sanctity of the organism so that it might reveal its true nature on its own terms, if so inclined? Would an awareness of this need enable its revelation? Perhaps the quality of our continuance depends on the seclusion of an organic self. *It may not be in our best interest to know everything.*

Despite everything that is known about consciousness, the essential element remains a mystery. Damasio (1999) writes: 'There is a mystery, however, regarding *how* images emerge from neural patterns. How a neural pattern *becomes* an image is a problem that neurobiology has not yet resolved.' Damasio goes on to say he is confident more discoveries will be made in this direction. Science may have its limitations. The way in which nervous activity 'becomes' non-material cognition is not known. Up until now, the *jump* between neurobiological activity and experience has proven to be 'uncatchable'. Perhaps this is nature's way of preserving our innocence.

Ultimately, consciousness is a movement in time with time. Without the flow of time there is no flow of consciousness. Ego consciousness interrupts organic consciousness (the proverbial stones in a stream). Time as an unfolding movement is inseparable from the fabric of consciousness, which is also an unfolding movement. Time and consciousness unfold as a unit. Consciousness continues to evolve as a movement and can be seen as an essential representation of creativity. We are *in creation* as consciousness unfolds. Consciousness, time and creation are a part of the same movement.

Using Consciousness

Whatever has been said regarding consciousness, however sophisticated our understanding of consciousness may be, how can we use our experience of it? As consciousness opens, we open, and we open to each other. A room full of people practising (something) together are sharing a collective consciousness highlighted by the practice. The feeling and the awareness are unmistakable. We enter into one another's field of consciousness and proceed from there. If, by going deeply into our personal tissues, we are revealing a consciousness less contaminated by conditioning, we are making a contribution to the quality of relationship.

A Body of Love

Where is the Love?

There is a feeling, a movement, akin to to love. It flows quietly, is not overly demonstrative, is texturally soft, and is supported by an inner strength. This feeling applies to the body and to a way of being.

In their teaching, spiritual guides draw attention to the elements that make up the positive and negative aspects of human behaviour. At the top of the list we can usually find love or, as it is often put, 'the question of love'. Love is the centre of gravity of human existence; we are programmed to love. Love is our true nature, waiting to greet us beneath the layers. Its derivatives, compassion, kindness, friendliness and tolerance lay beneath the surface. These feelings are good for us and release hormones that promote well-being and health.

For centuries, the yogis and Eastern practitioners have pointed the way to love, suggesting that love will arise if we go into ourselves and loosen our conditioning. We understand love through direct experience(s) and are aware of love if only through its absence. We know how elusive the condition of love can be. Our economic system and culture make it difficult for people to love one another. We are aware of the conflict between competition and compassion, between personal needs and social cohesion. Freud made some valid observations. He writes: 'So in every individual the two trends, one towards personal happiness and the other towards unity with the rest of humanity, must contend with each

other; so must the two processes of individual and of cultural development oppose each other and dispute the ground against each other' (1930).

In relation to self-interest, Erich Fromme writes: 'Individualism' which in its positive sense means liberation from social chains, means, in a negative sense, 'self-ownership' the right and the duty – to invest one's energy in the success of one's own person' (Source unknown). Freud states:

... this inclination towards an all embracing love of others and of the world at large is regarded as the highest state of mind of which man is capable. A love that does not discriminate seems to us to lose some of its own value, since it does an injustice to its object. And secondly not all men are worthy of love (Freud 1930).

However, the general condition of love is a feeling that takes everything in without discrimination and attachment. All things within one's field of consciousness, although some may be deemed unlovable, are within one's field of love. The feeling is personal to the one who loves simply because he or she has loving feelings. There is no effort; it is not a practice, although it may arise from certain practices.

We can and do live without love. When asked why people don't love each other, Krishnamurti simply replied, 'because they don't'! This observation did not deter him in his efforts to make a difference. Reich was more positive on the human condition. He writes: 'At the base of the neurotic mechanism, behind all the dangerous, irrational fantasies and impulses, I discovered a simple, self-evident, decent core. I found it without exception in every case where I was able to penetrate to a sufficient depth.'

Erich Fromme, like Freud, Krishnamurti and many others, suggested that our culture of 'having' dissipates the possibility of a culture of being, and that being is the gateway to more love (Fromme 1976). In *To Have or To Be*, he outlines a new blueprint for mankind based on less having and more being. Yoga has been advocating a similar blueprint for millennia.

Freud acknowledged yoga several times. He recounts how a respected friend assures him:

> ... the yogi by their practices of withdrawal from the world, concentrating attention on bodily functions, peculiar methods of breathing , are actually able to produce new sensations and diffuse feelings in themselves which he regards as regressions to primordial, deeply buried mental states. He [his friend] sees in them a physiological foundation, so to speak, of much of the wisdom of mysticism (Freud 1930).

Practice and Love

Can a system of body work mitigate conflict and encourage a generosity of feeling to surface, beyond the effects of endorphin release. This appears to be the case, but deeper changes may depend on the nature of the work. Loosening the physical tension within and between us makes a difference. The effect of tissue changes on 'how we are' is recognised by all types of body work. Whatever our physical condition, we can feel compassionate, but an improvement in physiology appears to enhance compassion. We are more giving when we feel good, and while we feel good.

If love is inherent, it is in the body. The mind might suggest and recognise feelings of love, but the feelings are released from the body. The body releases altruistic love in concert with the loosening of habit and conditioning. Body and breath work open a door, but are not an automatic guarantee of a 'more sustainable love'. Physiological changes promoting loving feelings need support from the additional practice of awareness in life. Our 'love interest' refers to an unsentimental, non-emotional being-in-love-ness that can exist in the background or foreground of awareness.

The Intelligence of Love

Love is an intelligence. Erotic love insures procreation, familial love provides nurture, and love across the board is an intelligent way to proceed, because it spreads out towards others, it unifies. *The General Theory of Love* (Lewis, Amini & Lannon, 2000) reminds us that all mammals have a 'limbic brain' lying above the non-emotional reptilian brain and beneath the rational cortex. Limbic organisation is concerned with caring for the young, bonding, and forming relationships; in a word, 'love'. The above volume suggests that although the neocortex is the most recent of the three areas, it is not the most advanced, implying that the limbic area is the most intelligent in terms of 'how we are' and the pleasure we derive from one another. The limbic area plays the essential role in social communication, caring, and awareness of others and their feelings. There is a 'love instinct' that arises from an evolutionary source. Mammals love their offspring and bond with each other, insuring the survival of the group. Human love may become buried by conditioning, but, as with one energy, and one consciousness, there is one condition of love. Love is organic; the organism loves.

Love Emerges in the Absence of its Detractors

The factors that impede deeper practice also inhibit emergent love. Negative tension, conditioning, habit and anxiety contrive to inhibit an outward movement of love. A major impediment is 'ownership'. Love is forthcoming when it is not *our love*, when we are simply in the 'love field'. A first step in inviting love is to sense the unlovable elements within us.

Nearly all detractors are stimulated by thought. When non-essential mental activity prevails, impediments seize their opportunity. 'In humans the neocortical capacity for thought can easily obscure other more occult mental activities' (Lewis, Amini & Lannon, 2000). The yogis have understood this for centuries, their entire remit being to loosen the grip of the cortex and allow love to emerge.

Krishnamurti suggests: 'love will come into being only when there is total self-abandonment' (Krishnamurti 1969). We need to drop a great deal before we can abandon the self that we know, even for a moment or two. But given the possibility, we need a strong base from which to let go. Abandonment needs support. One must feel anchored in oneself for authentic love to appear. Establishing a firm contact with the ground and cultivating a deep fluid strength of the spine provides such an anchor.

Love in Every Part

Oxytocin is the 'love hormone'. Life's most ancient process, reproduction, revolves around oxytocin. It is predominantly a female hormone, profuse in childbirth and orgasm, but men also produce and benefit from oxytocin. It has been around in animals before the arrival of mammals.

Acts of kindness towards others, prayer, compassion and gratitude produce oxytocin [the attitude of gratitude in practice]. Expressing feeling releases oxytocin [the feeling of expression itself]. Oxytocin is produced when we are inspired; this includes inspiration coming from another person's behaviour [bracketed text is mine] (Hamilton 2010).

Love hormones are secreted by glands, the limbic brain, the hypothalamus and the heart (the heart is truly an organ of love). Oxytocin is produced in nerve cells all over the body; receptors are found throughout the nervous system, in all tissues, fluids, and the space between the cells. It seems that the more scientists look for oxytocin sites, the more they find them. Love is in every part of us. A picture is emerging of oxytocin as a key component in a number of bodily systems, linking mind and body in a way never before understood (Hamilton 2010). This suggests that love hormones are found in spinal tissues and throughout the depth body. Feelings of love accompany sensations of fluid release, suggesting that cerebospinal fluid carries oxytocin.

Oxytocin is *the* relationship-enhancing hormone and is released during close and meaningful contact with others. It is profuse during biological functions demanding total surrender, such as orgasm or childbirth. Extending love to oneself also releases oxytocin. Oxytocin has a softening and melting effect on the body-mind. Oxytocin release is also connected to endorphin release, which draws us back time and again to the yoga experience by providing pleasurable sensations. 'Although endorphins are involved in the neurochemistry of bonding and love, the major player is probably oxytocin' (Young and Wang in Hanson 2009).

Deepening practice deepens this relationship and enhances the release of love hormones. The feeling of love during and following a class is well known. We love ourselves, our practice and the group. How long this lasts is variable, but every time we release the brakes on oxytocin we are resetting our potential for love across the board. Oxytocin is the hormone of brotherly love.

Practice, Love and Birth

Michel Odent, in *The Scientification of Love*, suggests that the prototype for all love is maternal love. His research points to the 'short, and yet critical period of time just after birth which has long-term consequences for our capacity to love' (Odent 1999). He suggests that interfering with this period has far-reaching consequences for mankind.

Michel Odent points out that during birth a cocktail of love hormones, important for birth and the period immediately following, are produced deeply inside the brain (hypothalamus and pituitary gland) and that their production can be inhibited by neocortical activity. In this respect, the two brains, ancient and recent, are at odds and the natural processes at work are suppressed. 'Any stimulation of the intellect in particular, can interfere with the process of labour' (Odent 1999). Michel Odent's research shows that neocortical activity inhibits the production of oxytocin, indicating that love flourishes during the reduction of thought. Overstimulation of the neo-cortex has the same effect on practice by inhibiting the activity of the deeper centres that promote love. Rational language (thought words), inappropriate or insensitive use of language in teaching, analysis, or even describing sensation to oneself, may contribute to inhibiting the primal centres that release love hormones.

There are clear correlations between how we practice and the physiology of birth. The more recent and the older brain have a tendency to oppose each other. We cannot control the ancient centres but we can modify the more recent ones. In some respects, the deep unfolding experience resembles a birth experience, although it is much less extreme. It can feel like the birth of unconditioned physiology expressing itself. Our highly developed intellect can be a handicap, letting it go enables profound results – more love.

We cannot change our birth experience but we can approach ourselves with more love. We can make love an immediate feature of practice. Love surfaces during an uncluttered relaxability in concert with inner strength and fluidity. Love arises when we are spontaneous. We should approach love's intelligence with the intelligence of love. We may court love through an Eastern or Western route but ultimately it comes from us. When we apply a loving attitude to the body, love comes back. Love comes when we give back to ourselves. The personal love that arises from love in practice can be a preliminary stage to the emergence of love generally.

The Breath of Love

Is love more prolific at the end of the exhalation, when we are deeply inside the spine, observing the seeds of expansion? 'There is not a single neurotic person who is capable of breathing out deeply and evenly in one breath' (Reich 1933). We may not see ourselves as neurotic, but our culture has neurotic tendencies. Neurosis inhibits an expression of love. Adjusting our breath, deepening its action, listening to its requirements might make a difference.

We can drop into a little more love at the end of an exhalation, as we receive an inhalation, where thought is unwelcome while feeling the deep movement of the breathing tissues inside us. Breathing and love are pleasurable sensations that can feed each other. Love comes with fluidity and softness. Delve into your love sites within your breath; sink into the unthinkingness of love.

Spirit of the Body

'I am a spiritual person.' What does that mean? Does it mean belief in a deity, a general feeling of goodwill to all, being a *nice* person, a tendency to introspect on a continual basis, a religious bent, a feeling of oneness with the universe? Interpretations of spirituality are taken up by the condition of love. Without love, all concepts of spirituality are dry and redundant.

Yoga-speak is full of spiritual reference. If we are going to go deeply into our tissues and ourselves, feelings and ideas related to spirituality will come up. If conditioning inhibits 'the spiritual experience', releasing our conditioning can deepen it. Spirituality is in our body, our flesh, breath and chemistry. We are born with it.

All aspects of our nature stem from an organic response to our environment. Spirituality may have been initially stimulated by a wonder of the outside world, but the feeling arises from the inside. Spirituality can be an idea, dependent upon an external agency, or it can be a total experience that includes the body. Alexander Lowen defined spirit as: 'The life force within an organism manifested in the self-expression of the individual' (Lowen 1958). Spirituality is physiological, arising from organic layers, but is recognised and distilled by conscious awareness. The combined effect of an ancient process and the realisational quality of the cortex provide spiritual insight.

The theological view suggests we are a response to God's will. The fact that spiritual feeling lies just beneath the surface is made evident by our responses in practice. On occasion, the first breath, the first responsive awakening, releases us into a spiritual experience. The Latin word for spirit, *spiritus/spirare*, means breath. When we are 'animated' we are full of life, spirited or inspired. Spirituality, like love and consciousness, is a feeling. Spirituality and love share the same chemistry; they arise from the same hormonal release and are activated as neocortical dominance retreats.

The underlying message of spiritual traditions is that we are capable of self-realisation, of being in the reality that lies beneath conditioning. Spirituality emerges as habitual tensions resolve and to the extent that our ego boundaries dissolve. When the neocortex takes a back seat, when it is toned down, we not only see the bigger picture more clearly, we feel it more deeply, we *are the bigger picture*. We may need spiritual thinkers if only to remind us to stop thinking.

Spirituality arises from the body. Jaap van der Wal suggests that spirituality begins at conception and is fostered throughout the early stages of embryological development (van der Wal 2003). Spiritual sensations are included in an original way of being; our spiritual nature has a physiological basis. Awakening our deeper physiology revitalises spiritual feelings.

Michel Odent suggests that our tendency towards spirituality may be released at the time of and just following birth, particularly if conditions are favourable. He gives the legend of the birth of Jesus as the perfect example. Mary gave birth in a stable, surrounded by mammals in an atmosphere of love, surrounded by creatures free from the interference of a neocortex (Odent 1999).

When you are in your spine, you could be releasing a spiritual dimension. The same goes for surfing the breath, blending with the ground, receiving fluid pulsations or being led by the sacrum. Wherever you go to in your body, the spirit is there. Iyengar's remark, typical of his genius at the time, 'how can you know God without the little toe', is a good example of every part of the body contributing to a peak (spiritual) experience (Iyengar 1987). The same can be said of each spinal articulation or tissue in the body. A new, deeper experience may be interpreted in a spiritual dimension. Spirituality arose from primal tissue. Going back into tissue reawakens a spiritual base.

An Organic Soul

The idea of a soul is based on organic properties. The word *'animate'* stems from the Latin anima, meaning breath, life, soul. To be animated is to be endowed with life, full of activity, spirited, inspired. Soul is also defined as our principle of life and our spiritual element, in contrast to physical substance, but arising from it. Early philosophers saw the soul as our animating source. *Animism* is the doctrine that the phenomena of animal life are produced by an immaterial anima or soul distinct from matter. Indian philosophy equates soul with consciousness and aligns it with 'universal consciousness'. Georg Feuerstein quotes Aristotle on soul: 'The soul is that by which we live, feel, or perceive, move and understand' (Feuerstein 1997). In other words, soul is everything.

We may *have* a soul, or we may *be a* soul. We can be soul-full. Someone can have soul in the sense that they have a resonant open-heartedness. To have soul implies that we have feeling. Soul, spirit and consciousness are part of the same movement, and their common denominator is energy. The more sensitive the organism becomes, the more obvious it is that this collective movement, this *one thing*, is an expression of sensitive aliveness. James Oschman points out that particular emotional states have been connected with measurable changes in the electrical energy spectrum of the heart and that the energy radiation of the heart is much greater than that of the brain (Oschman 2000). Love is literally positive energy.

Spirit and soul are words that describe aspects of existence. They are not separate from the body. We may invest more soul in the body or more body in the soul. Soul is in the tissues, in the texture of oneself, it manifests as an outward movement that arises from going inward. Experientially spirit and soul arise into awareness from the deep organic tissue that feeds consciousness. Spirit and soul arise from the involuntary aspects of the organism. We don't *do* spirit and soul; they emerge as a way of being. The energy that moves outward from within has a component that could be called spirit, soul or heart and soul, derivatives of inherent love. 'The embryo is not *getting* a soul, it *is* soul as well' (van der Wal 2003).

Love is a Movement

The entire body-mind radiates an all-encompassing feeling as a consequence of deep practice. The ego softens and consciousness opens up to make way for a spontaneous radiation that is best described as love. This love is personal, but has no target and may feel oceanic or universal. It is as if one enters into a *field of love* that has

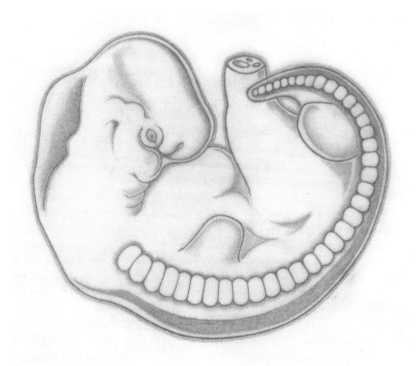

Figure 18.1

A soul expressing itself.

always been present. There is no need for a specific focus of love; everything is included. Love, spirituality and soul are one movement in time with time and demonstrate the polarity between 'our depth' and the infinite space around us. The condition of 'more love' is not emotional, although it does emote (move out from within), but is a flow of feeling through and from the body.

Love's Sensations

Feelings of your connection to the ground, the breath, the enormous expansion from within contain an element of love. Love comes with sensations of softness, fluidity and space. Releasing tension from the surface of the body, reinforcing the spine's vitality, centring, grounding, and paying quiet attention are acts of love.

It seems that oxytocin is more effective when released rhythmically, in a succession of fast pulsations (Odent 1999). This observation is compatible with the experience in practice of the involuntary pulsations and waves that course through the body and provide us with sensations of emergent love.

Original Love

There is a difference between loving your practice and practising with love. Do you practise with love or without love? There is a clear dividing line; we either do or we don't. It takes a small adjustment of consciousness, a gentle mental shift, working with soft attention, to encourage the body to reveal its love to us. The love that comes is usually a peak experience and then it drops. But we learn from it, remember and return to it. As time goes by a positive tendency may become more established.

Depth could reveal a self-serving aggressive nature. Freud took a bleak view: we have unavoidable aggressive tendencies, we are full of fear, the nemesis of love, love arises when it suits us. Aggression might be called for under certain circumstances but does not arise naturally when we get to the bottom of things; but love does, perhaps because we are reproducing womb-like and early bonding sensations. Positive feelings enhance love. When we feel warm inside, soft, fluid, flowing, pulsatile, and supported by the earth, the mind and emotions take part. When we pare back to basic organic function, love reinstates itself. A deeper practice might reveal a deeper, more enduring love.

Involuntary movements stimulate involuntary love. As involuntary movement wells up from the body, it brings an involuntary expression of loving feelings. Love arises of its own accord, because it is an original state. It arises when we 'feel free from ourselves'. This observation acknowledges the old Indo-European word for love, seen in Sanskrit, meaning 'free'.

As the original body awakens, cutting through the layers surrounding it, it pushes love to the surface. Your body expresses love and your mind accepts. The combination of love, arising from ancient structures, and its recognition by the neocortex gives love its power. When we can acknowledge feelings of love, when they are in conscious awareness, our perception of them enhances their presence. 'Love is not a thing that one can have, but a *process*, an inner activity that one is the subject of. I can love, I can *be* in love, but in loving, I have . . . nothing. In fact, the less I have, the more I can love (Fromme 1976).

Biological science identifies the molecular activity producing feelings of love but cannot bridge the gap between the chemistry and the experience of love; it remains a mystery. Love remains a mysterious experience. We may *know* about the neuro-hormonal aspects of love, but *when* we love, information *about* love seems superfluous and is an avoidance of love itself. When love is activated we feel it everywhere. It permeates our being and our world. Theories regarding personal experience are plentiful. Love is no exception. Moment-to-moment experience moves, changes its texture, intensity and content, in myriad ways. If there is an authority that might understand or follow a loving feeling, it is the experiencer. We ourselves are the authority on love. We are the authors of the nature of, and the relationship between, our physical sensations, breathing, tissue texture, involuntary behaviour, and how we are affected by, and act on them. We move through soft tissue, fluid, articular space, emotion, intuition and insight, into heart and soul.

Behaviour

Behaviour Defined

Changes in physiological behaviour can change behaviour generally. We may or may not feel a need for, or anticipate, modifications in behaviour, but they occur spontaneously. The organism sponsors a more intelligent self, giving us a taste of, and opportunity for, shifts in the way we conduct ourselves internally and externally.

We *are* behaviour. Evolutionary and embryological development are behavioural processes. The sperm cell seeking the egg cell, the unfolding of the blastula within the uterus and the expression of foetal limbs are behaviours. The organism is a behaviourist upon which we impose our personal patterns of behaviour. 'The embryo performs or exhibits gestures and motions; it performs actions by its growing and changing Being (or Becoming). This means: an embryo exhibits (growing) behaviour (van der Wal 2003).

All activity is behaviour, whether it refers to personal expression or to organic expressions of life. Personal behaviour is defined by the English Oxford Dictionary as 'The manner of conducting oneself'. Organic behaviour is described by Collins as (a) 'The aggregate of all the responses made by an organism in any situation' and (b) 'A specific response of a certain organism to a specific stimulus or group of stimuli, or manner of acting or controlling oneself.' The roots of the word *behaviour* stem from the old English *behabban*, and from the Latin *habere*, meaning habit. The French word *avoir*, meaning 'to have', has the same roots. These definitions relate behaviour to 'having habitual personal conduct and on the species driven level to survival in our habitat'. Primal behaviour is generally uniform, while personal behaviour is open to modification. We can describe types of behaviour but behaviour itself is indescribable. At best, we can describe our experience of behaviour, which is also a form of behaviour. Experience is behavioural.

Behaviour and Awareness

All expression is behavioural. Spinal waves are a form of behaviour. Spinal curves have developed to accommodate an original behaviour needed to stand on two legs. We did not begin life on land with secondary lumbar and cervical curves but unself-consciously grew into them as they grew into us. The unfoldment of young organisms from a centre, from a central nervous system, from a respiratory diaphragm and spine, is a form of behaviour. As practice deepens, we enhance an unfoldment of energy, forming the basis for all expression. Unimpeded unfoldment taps into primal behaviour and passes through personal patterns of behaviour. Habit and conditioning make way for the emergence of original behaviour.

Behaviour can be divided into Six Categories

1. *Energetic vibrational behaviour lying beneath all activity* — a feature of all organisms that can be experienced as aliveness, streaming or currents,

2. *Involuntary organic behaviour* — the basic behaviour of the species as energy acts on structure — experienced as pulsations, waves, and fluidity, the small movements,

3. *Involuntary mechanical behaviour* — such as articulatory activity, skeletal movement, and the tensional activity of muscle tissue and fascia in response to gravitation and breathing, experienced as myofascial — skeletal activity,

4. *Voluntary organic and mechanical behaviour* — arising from the conscious will to act and react in response to internal needs and the dictates of the environment, experienced as movements that includes involuntary sensations; larger movements underpinned by smaller ones,

5. *Personal patterns of body/mind behaviour* — in response to cultural, social and familial (and possibly genetically inherited factors), some of which occurs beneath conscious experience, inhibit the above behaviours, and may restrain organic behaviour,

6. *Additional personal patterns of body/mind behaviour* — relating to individual history and life's events beyond social, cultural and familial conditioning, which contains conditioned patterns lying beneath conscious experience and may further constrain organic behaviour.

All behaviours are superimposed upon their predecessor(s). The most basic are dulled to awareness by the more recent conditioned patterns. In principle and practice, we can to some extent dissolve the conditioning, bring the underlying activity in to conscious awareness, and clear inhibitive patterns. In so doing, the deeper organic and energetic properties realise a more prolific expression. Underlying activity emerges energetically, organically and mechanically.

Personal Behaviour

Mammals behave in accordance with the general behaviour of their species. Behaviour becomes more diverse as we move up the evolutionary scale. The increase in size of the neocortex, its sensitivity and imaginative range, enables a sophisticated variety of behaviours. Knowing what might or could happen provides fertile ground for all kinds of behaviour.

Positive aspects of personal creative behaviour emerge through the neocortex, but we pay the price. Awareness of our mortality, vulnerability, and *our behaviour*, invites a wide ranging conduct, some of which may be classified as neurotic (Horney 1937). External behaviour is driven by the intensity, rate, and content of internal behaviour. Catching a glimpse of each other's inner thoughts, perceptions and feelings, might be unhelpful in relationships. Experience shows that we become more aware of our internal behavior as the primal behavior underpinning it begins to surface.

Thought, Emotion and Behaviour

Thought arising from the mind provokes imagination and arouses emotion, which stimulates a substantial proportion of our behaviour. Preparing for the next thing, and for the future, is essential for survival and creativity, but in a negative light thought invites fear of what might happen, or of what might be repeated. Antonio Damasio writes: 'In effect, normal human behaviour exhibits a continuity of emotions induced by a continuity of thoughts' (Damasio 2000).

Behaviour is coloured by experience with an emotional content. Emotional expression, whether released or not, is physiological. Holding back expression is another form of expression. The way we move, our physical behaviour, can be an indication of internal behaviour, whether consciously experienced or unavailable to awareness through conditioning. This was particularly clear in 'mental institutions' but can be seen in many people; we all have our patterns. Many people are unaware of their underlying physical behaviour in daily life. A shoulder forward may be a behaviour hidden from awareness until pointed out, and may contain an aspect of personal history. We use the outer layers to contain the expression within.

Behaviour and Tension

Species-driven behaviour contains little if any conflict other than a resistance imposed by more recent layers. Personal behaviour may be full of conflict. All behaviour is internal and becomes externalised spontaneously unless consciously censored by personal adjustment or constraint. However we may appear outwardly, we generally know the content and intensity of our internal behaviour, but not always, and it may take a therapist to point out or confirm what we suspect or remain unaware of. We may censor external behaviour, but much of our internal behaviour cannot be censored. We are masterful at not saying what we feel or think, and for good reason. Having the faculty of censorship does nothing to placate the ever-shifting and unpredictable content of internal behaviour. In effect, a tension exists between what we keep to ourselves and what we show.

Freud's observation that behaviour is generally caught between instinctual drives and cultural and social codes of conduct (Freud 1930) not only prevails, but has provided the basis for yoga practice for many centuries. We are driven by personal needs but have a need to 'fit in' and be accepted by the group. Consequently, we temper our basic drives and impulses. Although motivated independently, we are bound by a conflicting need for interdependence. However singular we may feel, we follow the herd. Many personal growth activities address the tension that contains basic impulses, but without necessarily carrying them through to what could be an inappropriate conclusion. Yoga, on the other hand, was intended to convert the energy of basic drives into a personal awakening. We may or may not use practice in this way, but in general terms deep work sublimates drives inappropriate for

expression while enabling the manifestation of acceptable ones.

Polarised Behaviour

Whether driven by circumstance, conditioning or an expression of life, all behaviour is physiological. Behaviour that rises into awareness is contained within a broader field of behavioural activity. Behaviour presents a polarity, with the organism and its expressive simplicity at one end and the neocortex with its individual complexity, restlessness, creativity and knowledge at the other end. Between organic and mental behaviour lies mechanical behaviour. By attending to skeletal configurations through exploratory movement and breathing, we can satisfy organic behaviour, enhance personal behaviour and bring more balance to their polarity.

Sensitivity and Behaviour

Yoga observes internal and external behaviour but focuses predominately on the internal. The introspective element of yoga is concerned with restoring internal behaviour to a satisfactory condition. We might address ourselves by sinking back into the primal behaviour of the body and bring it to the forefront of awareness. With the addition of awareness, we can, in part, bring our involuntary behaviour to the surface. Yoga makes us more sensitive to our physiology, state of mind, our internal and external behaviour, and the quality of relating. We become more sensitive to spinal nuances, pulsations, tensional interactions, and the compulsion to override or withdraw.

Our conditioning is not our fault, but we are responsible for our behaviour *when we notice it*. It is surprising how many people are relatively unaware of their internal conduct. Once the door begins to open, as we hone away at depth sensitivity, change occurs on other levels. Primal movement pushes personal conflict before it, and as a consequence also unveils the positive aspects of spontaneity which include friendliness, kindness and joy, all expressions of a relaxed and contented organism.

The remit of yoga is to encourage flow between layers. The mind penetrates the body and the body reveals itself to the mind. We move inwards from the outside and move outwards from within, inviting a behavioural harmony. The agenda of the yogis was to transcend conditioned behaviour, and move beyond conflict created by divisions. We do this continually as our work deepens and we notice and cultivate the accumulative effects.

Ethical Behaviour

It is normal and part of the process for teachers and students to bond. We work and share insights together. As we move through deeper layers, we can be exposed to situations needing discretion and sensitivity. Any lines to be drawn are our responsibility. Krishnamurti was particularly sensitive regarding his position and would 'rewind' his day, looking for ways in which he might have put things differently. Behaviour is an essential meditation. Common sense dictates an awareness of conduct as working with others provides a fertile arena for projection and transference. Students are grateful for good experiences, for their progress and at times may feel vulnerable. It is a responsibility. Yoga is ethical, but practice does not necessarily guarantee immunisation against pitfalls. The deeper we go, the greater the potential for releasing old patterns, but as we unfold with sensitivity, behaviour tends to adjust itself to all situations, if and when they arise. Gravity, depth of action and soft fluid strength are effective levellers, adding a valuable touch of sobriety to the joy of new discoveries.

Deep work changes behaviour from below up, and from within out. The physiological changes that accompany free expression enhance temperament, mood, timing, responsiveness and intelligence. There is always a circumstance waiting in the wings.

Beyond Practice

Beyond Practice

Physiological totality is the precursor to the 'one with everything feeling'.

This is a practical book and constantly refers to practice. The word 'practice' from the Latin *practica* means to 'practise familiar or practical knowledge', the implication being that practice concerns something that is known. Styles of practice are concretions containing ideas about how practice should be, feel and look. But we are given the opportunity to move beyond practice, which is a construct, a device used, to move into something more open than our habitual body-minds. Practice at first deepens our personal sense of self. It gives us a base from which to move beyond. If there is little there to begin with, we have nowhere to go, at least nowhere in a positive sense. We find a balance between a strong self and freedom from oneself and move between the two.

Young mammals play at activities they will eventually need for survival. The developing embryo and foetus appear to practise movements that might be forerunners of those needed after birth. These movements might satisfy a need for expression. Perhaps the organism is self-practicing.

We must start somewhere. Transcending established patterns does not just happen. It is unlikely that practice will make us perfect because there is no perfection in the act of practicing. Practice is the way in but not the thing.

In whatever way we *use* practice, we pass *through* it. Slipping into the underlying nature of the organism moves us beyond practice and into the beyond-ness feeling. As we proceed, we realise shifts in how we are. We move beyond a consolidated sense of self. We have the personal experience of being beyond personal experience.

Original Yoga

Yoga is original in that it draws on the personal inquiry of each practitioner. The original yoga experience had no idea of yoga, but drew on organic sensations from its evolutionary past moving into and through the present. What seems to us to be beyond is original because it is beyond the neocortex.

Moving beyond takes us into something more spacious, relaxed, awake, and more connected to our depth and to the world/universe around us. We remember the experience. Although some spiritual teachers recommend un-experiencing as an ideal state, we cannot learn from an un-recordable experience but might feel refreshed by it. Being without oneself, even momentarily, has beneficial effects.

The physical work acts as a passage, an ultimate door to an alternative experience. How do you feel as you are swept up in a tide of tensional release, empty the last vestige of exhalation, as sensation, emotion and thought fuse, as you let go of the familiar sense of *yourself*? Where do you go and how do you feel when you come back?

Beyond-ness

Transcendence is not an unobtainable state. We transcend continually in our thoughts and feelings. We may knowingly transcend desires, regrets, disappointments, impatience, resentment, and so on. Every small containment, each letting go, or adjustment of an impulse is a transcendence. Spiritual guides appear to live in a continuum of transcendence, a culture of allowing. Transcendence can be seen as an Eastern ideal that subscribes to the possibility of moving beyond oneself, but at its simplest is a tempering of internal behaviour as a consequence of attention and recognition.

Transcendence, like consciousness and the energy that drives it, is a movement. Transcendence involves being awake enough to *field* one's reactions as they come up. Moving beyond is slipping out of our conditioning into something that feels spacious, relaxed, awake and connected to our deeper selves and to the world. Beyond is original because it is beyond the habitual neocortex and free from conditioning. Beyond-ness, in its purest sense, is consciousness free from thought, recognition and registration.

Passing through the Body

As we practice, we transcend voluntary activity and move into involuntary activity. The exchange between voluntary and involuntary action comes and goes, gradually giving way to involuntary activity as the body takes over. The physical work acts as a passage through ourselves. The feeling of total physiological activity enables us to pass into the 'one with everything feeling'. Moving from skin to spine, from the space around us to deep inner space, takes us through and beyond ourselves.

Every time we resist an impulse to draw the inhalation, wait for the spine to move before moving, or allow mental interference to pass by, we are transcending impatience, control, wanting and expectation. When your allow your body to take you, you transcend fear of abandonment. When you accept the primal movement

of the spine and relinquish ownership of your tissues, you transcend yourself.

When we are supported by the ground, when the physiology that we inhabit expresses itself freely and with minimal interference, the opportunity arises for change on all levels. When the entire body feels like an integrated organ, we might experience its connection to everything beyond it. We can perceive the earth as an organ with ourselves as organs within it or, to go further, the universe as an organ with ourselves the atomic particles.

'Merging with the Cosmos implies complete surrender to one's bodily sensations, as though nature were simply flowing through unimpeded' (Baker 1967).

Beneath the Barrier

Beyond lies beneath and within, manifesting as energetic activity arising upwards and outwards through the system and, passing through our external familiar self. Beyond is beneath tissue, the breath, spinal awakening and mental patterning. Beyond lies beneath practice, and beyond ideas about being beyond.

The neocortex presents a barrier between the inner and outer worlds, between the deep body and surrounding space. As the texture of the brain softens in concert with the flowing fluidity of the body, the barrier melts, the inner dance reaches out beyond encapsulation. Michel Odent writes:

Our new brain supports the concepts of time, space and boundaries, including the limits of our life span. These concepts define our sense of identity, which only develops in infancy once the human neocortex is sufficiently developed, and seems to correspond to that stage when the child is able to recognise herself in a mirror. When we are wide awake we see the universe from a neocortical perspective. *The older sub-neocortical structures on the other hand provide us with our sense of being part of a whole. They support another reality – one that transcends the concepts of space and time and boundaries [italics author]* (Odent 1999).

When the neocortex is quiet, in the background, and on occasion non-existent, the energy from below moves upward, releasing the grip of the upper layers. Feelings of beyond-ness come from below the summit of familiar experience. When the approach is favourable, the body-mind slips easily into beyond-ness and takes the opportunity to sink beneath conditioning. Returning to sensation as a meditation gives the mind to the body. Chip Hartranft, in his book on the Sutras of Patanjali, writes:

Thought, emotion and feeling like a self are all constructive in nature and arise against a background of sensory inputs. When we give attention to the sensory field and keep it there we become more sensitive to the most subtle emergences of thought, feeling and I'ness. This constructive activity then begins to stand out and can be recognised for what it is, a mental product that is conditioned, impersonal and mandatory – when the will not to react is applied to the sensory field from moment to moment the self's possessive grip on the percept is loosened and broken (Hartranft 2003).

Where do we go to when we go?

Where do we go when we go beyond? We obviously have not *gone anywhere*. Where does beyond-ness come from? The deeper we venture in, the further we go out. The changes that arise from going inward remind us that we are *one with everything*. We penetrate our physiology to embody this realisation.

It's not surprising that we have oceanic and universal feelings. We came out of the ocean and are part of the universe. Dissolving the barriers between ourselves and our origins brings up these feelings. Sensations of unlimited expansion are 'original sensations' contained within genetic memory and perceived by personal experience. Our deep energy is attracted to universal energy, the fluid body is attracted to the moon and stars, and the spine dances with gravity.

The deeper we go into our physical substance, the more connected we feel to the bigger picture. The more subservient the cortex becomes to the deeper body, the more expansive we feel as we dissolve the barrier between our inner and outer worlds. We enter the microcosm of ourselves (inner cosmos), which gives the feeling of an intimate connection to the cosmos at large.

'If our body is the matter to which our consciousness applies itself it is coextensive with our consciousness, it comprises all we perceive, it reaches the stars' (Feuerstein 2003).

It seems to me that as we release the tensions of 'holding it together' we revert to a state where the ego-body existed without the inhibitory influence of the ego-self. 'The feelings of ego-maturity developed out of this original unlimited sense of being 'one with everything' (Freud 1930).

Georg Feuerstein writes:

Perhaps when we have come to fully appreciate the fact that cosmos and brain are of one mould, we will also realise that we do not have to spend billions of dollars to explore distant planets or travel to the nearest star, but that we can be psychocosmonauts, as earlier yogis were. As the ancients knew, microcosm and macrocosm are one and the same. It looks increasingly so (Feuerstein 2003).

Science examines the nature of the universe and our part in it through theories arising from the general theory of relativity and quantum mechanics. In scientific terms, the general theory of relativity describes the macro structure of the universe from a few miles to millions upon millions of miles, while quantum mechanics describes the extremely small-scale micro phenomena to within millionths of an inch (Stephen Hawking 1988). This may resonate with yoga practitioners. We feel the grand scheme of things connecting to inner space when we release the *habit of us*. The deeper we go, the more out there we feel. Infinity feels internal and external, interfaced by an ever-decreasing physical density.

Expansion and Density

The 'interior' of atoms and the 'space' between atoms are a vast emptiness, and yet our sensory experience confronts us with objects that appear stubbornly solid (Feuerstein 1997).

The yoga experience is based upon the relationship between density or attraction and expansion or distraction. Physicists suggest that stars constantly move away from each other but at the same time are being slowed down by gravity (Stephen Hawking 1988). It is proposed that an original universe had such extreme density or contraction that it responded by exploding into expansion. The universe is expanding by between 5 and 10 per cent every thousand million years and will expand for ever.

Georg Feuerstein quotes the British physicist Harold Schilling: 'For him, and many other physicists, the universe has not only spatial extension but also depth upon depth, or what he calls "interiority"' (Schilling in Feuerstein 2003). One could say that the human body expands from depth and condensation, representing a microcosmic version of universal dynamics.

Feelings of density and expansion are physiological and felt in the body. The deeper we investigate density the more we expand. It feels that by going inwards, into the body, condensing the molecules of the self, we open in all directions, an expansion of infinite vastness, of out there-ness. When the body is in expansion, *it takes the mind with it*. Opening the body empties consciousness.

The new physics has furnished us with an exhilarating image of the universe and thus of ourselves. The cosmos is now conceptualised as an infinite ocean of energy that is organised into extraordinarily complex patterns, of which the human body-mind is just one configuration of energy (Feuerstein 1997).

Time

We are more conditioned by time than any other single factor. Embryological time, foetal time, growth time, lifetime, historical and evolutionary time conspire to give us a finite view of time. A beginning and end to everything. The yogis would say we are *of* time, an insight that becomes more apparent as we continue to delve into the potential of what we do. Our attitude to time colours beyond-ness.

How do you experience time in practice? As a measurement, a movement, a feeling, or all of these things. Time is the primary movement of life, the original factor in existence. All biological activity is secondary to the movement of time because time was here before

we were. We are a product of time. Human evolution is an animate expression of time.

Self-Time

The use of time as a measurement is essential for organising our lives. In one way or another, we continually refer to the past and future. Aside from using time as measurement, our conditioning is tied to time because of the past. In life we cannot avoid divisionary time but we can in practice, should it prove counterproductive. When we get *caught* by time, we exercise control, we control the practice, time controls us. There is no freedom in what just happened and what might happen.

Stephen Hawking says: 'In the theory of relativity there is no unique absolute time, but instead each individual has his own personal measure of time that depends on where he is and how he is moving' (Hawking 1988). All time can only be experienced personally, but this does not alter our sense of *being* in a time that is beyond us. 'Self-time' and beyond self-time are personal experiences reflecting another polarity. Being weighted towards self-time, in practice, inhibits the reorganisation of personal patterns. Moving beyond self-time frees consciousness for a deeper and more fluid body-mind sensitivity.

Original Time

No experience is impersonal. Only the experience of no experience is impersonal but cannot exist as experience because there is no self to experience it. The experiencer can, however, unify with the experience. The organism has no idea of time; it is in time with time; it is not separated from time by registering time. *Being* in time with universal time takes us out of ourselves and takes the self out of us.

Universal time has no agenda but simply is. We can learn from the innocence of time; it does not divide itself; we do that. Stephen Hawking (1988) suggests the possibility of time beginning with the beginning of the universe, that is, if it ever began at all. He writes: 'One could say: the boundary condition of the universe is that it has no boundary. The universe would be completely self-contained and not effected by anything outside itself. It would be neither created nor destroyed. It would just BE.' Hawking's proposal resonates with our experience of *being*. Time is something we feel as a component of the general feeling of being. We can factor time into our general sense of the bigger picture.

Physiological Time

When the deep body moves involuntarily, without the mind's direction, we might be reverting to a time when movement was spontaneous and reflexive. It feels as if an ancient period reveals itself through the body, a period when we were an integral part of the whole, a time when we were unaware of time.

Hawking suggests that the realisation of time was instrumental in the early development of consciousness (Hawking 1988). Because consciousness is rooted in the body we can appreciate time as a physical sensation. Psychological time follows physiological time, which reveals itself through sensation; time is a physical feeling.

Physiological time is an integral part of the movement of awareness and our sense of being. Body time has no self-history but has a biological history reflected in our evolutionary development. Molecular information conveys the movement of the past flowing into the future as we continue to evolve. As soon as we try to get back to where we were, or want something to happen, we trap ourselves in self-time.

In practice, awareness, movement and aliveness move in time with time. Time is a feeling passing through our tissues, bones, liquidity and awareness. All sensation moves with time because sensation is a movement; it does not stand still. Universal time and self-time are in the body, universal time more so because we are a synthesis of universal constituents. Universal time is the void from which all things materialised. To whatever extent we are conditioned by self-time, universal time is more powerful.

Time Movement

George F.R. Ellis, in his paper 'The Flow of Time', says:

The most important property of time is that it unfolds. The present is different from both the past and future, which in turn are completely different from each other, the past being fixed and the future changeable. The present is the instant of transition between the two states. The time that is the present at this instant will be in the past at the next instant. This process of coming into being rolls on in an immutable way: while we can influence what happens in time, we cannot influence the way that time itself progresses on (Ellis 2008).

In this respect 'there is no now', only movement. 'For us (physicists) the distinction between past, present and future is an illusion, albeit a stubborn one.' (Albert Einstein, source unknown).

Gebser writes on Aristotle:

He proceeds from the point of view that the 'now' does not exist since it is at once the end of the past and the beginning of the future. Consequently he considers it to be merely a kind of 'in between' which interrupts or interlinks as a fixed point in space and time without beginning or end (Gebser 1945).

The movement of time does not settle upon things, it passes through mental activity connected to past or potential events. Gebser states: 'The fourth dimension is time freedom — in its conscious form — original archaic time freedom brought into consciousness, i.e. we become aware of time freedom' (Gebser 1945). True freedom is freedom from time. The body-mind unfolds; this is our experience. The simple experience of time is movement. Time is the essential movement of life.

We feel it in ourselves. Time emanates from the body as primal activity taking us 'back to a time' when we had no idea of time. The past flows through now into the future. I might be moving towards a future result based on past experience. This might be necessary, but once I am there, I have no need of the past or the future. My body unfolds between both into the movement of now.

Thought and Time

You can think about the past and the future but the thinking itself takes place in the present. Current thinking is *now*, whether we refer to the past or future. You could say that the mind is always in the present because thinking about the past or future is happening in the present — *the function of the mind is in the present but the present is a movement*.

'The conscious mind can also think forward and backward in time, while the subconscious mind is always operating in the present' (Lipton 2005). The truth is that *we are always in the now, but as a movement* — to whatever extent we may refer to the past or project into the future, we are in the now while referring to past and future.

Jean Gebser writes on time:

The events of tomorrow are always ideally present today. Tomorrow is nothing other than a today which is not yet acute, i.e. is still latent. Every manifestation of our own lives inevitably contains the sum of what is past as well as what is to come ... The present is not identical with the moment but is the undivided presence of yesterday, today and tomorrow which in a consciously realised actualisation can lead to a presentation which encompasses origin as an ineradicable present (Gebser 1945).

Feelings of timelessness indicate that we are in time with time. We sense time as a movement that flows with and through consciousness. As depth work reveals ancient properties, the past moves through the present into the future which is the moving sensation of now. The length of a breath is irrelevant.

East and West

Yoga masters throughout the ages have acknowledged that regardless of culture, yoga lies beneath all forms and patterns of human conditioning. Each of us contains the yoga seed. The West has embraced the physical and the mindfulness aspects of yoga, but hesitates over a more profound possibility. A deeper transcendence may be unpalatable for Western culture and its appetites.

The common ground between Eastern and Western practitioners outweighs their differences. The Eastern body-mind gravitates more deeply and is more accepting of the universal scheme of things. But East and West are open to deep body sensations, have the same respiratory apparatus, the same number of spinal vertebrae, and the potential to open up on all levels. The ego and the physiology of tension are the same East or West. We spring from a common evolutionary and embryological source. On a deep level, there are no differences between Eastern and Western practitioners. Beneath our cultural cloaks we are the same. We all move and feel from the same place, and have evolved upward and outward from our centre.

The Eastern mind may have tuned into consciousness in a particular way, but, we all have conscious awareness and turbulent minds. East or West, the human condition is one of being conditioned.

Interpretations may differ between individuals of the same culture. What feels like an expansion of the soul to some may feel like opening of the fascia lining the chest to others. Primal experiences might carry a spiritual element to some and anatomical insight to others, or both. As the primal body pushes outward and upward to engage the interest of the cortex, the stimulation may herald any number of individual interpretations linked to cultural and personal expression.

East and West have had an interest in the nature of consciousness, but through different routes, the Western interest coming later. The East sought and fostered a universal experience through yoga and meditation, while the West sought an understanding of our madness and confusion through analysis. Western analysis dissected personal history while yoga passed through and beyond it and, although acknowledging the impediments along the way, gave little attention to family history.

Freud and his contemporaries were interested in *what* lie beneath the self, in terms of unconscious, repressed conflicts. The East had always seen the undercurrents as irrelevant and superficial, pointing to a universal consciousness at a deeper level, from which a pure and unconditioned realisation sprang. Their approach sought an awakening that had been obscured by our 'sleeping state'. Their point was to remove impediments without analysis. Western investigation focused on the *content* of repressed material.

Countless publications on yoga, by Eastern and Western authorities, many following ancient guidelines, all ultimately speaking from their own experience, suggest that the yoga experience involves relaxation combined with wakefulness. This experience contains feelings of stillness, emptiness, flow, lightness detachment, connectedness to the environment, understanding, unknowing, beyond-ness and love, potentially crowned by a little bliss or joy.

In Western yoga, inquiry has attracted anatomical considerations and drawn from the research and experience of 'bodywork' while in the East there is more focus on the energetic and spiritual aspects. East and West continue to study the effects and benefits of mindfulness, the easily accessible essence of yoga. It is accepted in the West that our understanding may be limited in comparison to the realisations put forward by Eastern practitioners. This is reflected in our attraction to India and Tibet. Easterners traditionally had a tendency to value their universal origin while undervaluing their individuality. Westerners, on the other hand, tend to invest more in their individuality while undervaluing their universal origins.

Krishnamurti suggested throughout his lifetime of teaching that we should not get caught up in the past or in systems, that we could 'get there' right now. He recommended vigilance, attention and focus on what 'is'. When asked by a student if his many years of teaching had been understood by many, he is reported to have replied, 'perhaps by one or two'. Osho's comment on Krishnamurti's message was that he did not give people a door, give them something to do, such as meditation, as a means of entry. This may be so, but he delivered a valuable message with extraordinary insight. In terms of finding it in oneself and for oneself, Krishnamurti was original.

Whatever the culture, going into ourselves is a personal enquiry. There can be as much interest in the East or West in changing patterns. Practices from the East have come West but the West is also developing its own ways of approaching personal growth, some of which are based on traditional Eastern practices, and some which are not. There are only so many ways to breath, so many positions and meditations. The organism has no interest in cultural difference or similarities but seeks an expression common to all. This expression can be a profound and enlightening experience when we do the work. An Eastern and Western practitioner in the same room, with the intention of awakening the organism may have the same experience.

And Now

It will be interesting to see how yoga will disseminate into mainstream life as time goes by. Georg Feuerstein points out that the practice of yoga goes back 5,000 years, translating into about 200 generations, while the history of the United States goes back about ten generations. He goes on to say:

Yoga has definitely come West. Now the challenge before us is to unlock its full potential, when we are willing to practice it in *depth*. I like to contemplate the possibility of a future civilization that lives by such lofty yogic principles as non-harming, kindness, tolerance, cooperation, forgiveness, contentment, peace, and genuine happiness [italics author] (Feuerstein 2003).

At the last count, it has been estimated that in the United States yoga has become a $7 billion a year industry, and is predicted to reach $8 billion dollars by 2017 (*The Economist* November 2014).

Communication

What We Do

A group unfolds and, finding its point of release, realises its inner strength and deep fluidity. Everyone begins to move in the same way as physiology speaks from an ancient time.

Due to its nature, Yoga is unteachable; it is a personal experiment based on each practitioner's experience. We provide a structure within which students can learn for themselves. We can teach the framework and bring students towards the experience. Frameworks are dry; experience is rich. We cannot accompany students into their deep tissues or control their sensations, and would not want to. To do so would empower the teachers while disempowering the students. Introducing students to a *deeper creature* through the realisation of their own depth is beyond technique.

The word education comes from the Latin word *educare*, meaning to draw out, in other words, to draw out something that exists, draw out an original body free from habit and conditioning. To draw out we have to go in. We can't directly teach primal movement but we can guide others inward so that they may draw it out for themselves. Students are empowered as they discover the freedom and strength that lies within them. But we can come as close as we can to providing them with an experience. Experientially focused communication is teaching at its best; it is a challenge and a skill.

Each of us has our personal way of teaching. It is as individual as our own practice. Guiding others into

deep work is no different. As your own practice deepens, your language and style of communication changes spontaneously. Profound communicability arises by itself. People may come to you because you work deeply. If they have heard about your work, and the level at which you work is unexpected, they will have an opportunity they had not anticipated.

The Individual within the Group

Everyone holds a personal pattern. We are inviting a group of individuals to pass through their individuality and open up to 'what lies beneath'. Individual patterns drop away as groups find a common expression. Although the timing and speed of activity may differ between individuals, the movement follows a similar pathway without stylisation! Appealing to individuality with word language satisfies the ego and it will step aside more readily. One's choice of words may have different effects on different people. Targeting group depth may find new places for each person, but a common thread emerges.

We teach from our own practice and from what we see and sense in the group. The more we introduce a style or method, the further we move away from a common truth. Teaching involves communicating our experience to others by imparting *our* depth to *their* potential depth. Reversing spinal curves or bathing in fluid release becomes a group experience. With this in mind, each of us develops our own way of communicating.

The Product

Teaching methods or styles bring expectations. It is worth reminding the group that a *style* might give an excuse for 'not finding it in oneself'. We may work methodically but physiology has no method. Given a method, it should appeal to natural physiological behaviour and assist the body in enhancing its inherent tendencies. Prospective students may need an idea of what to expect. If you are someone who advertises or markets yourself, you might need a product. You could try the product of no product. Once new students are on site, the work will speak for itself.

Inspiration

Two fundamental attributes are needed to teach well: the ability to communicate and inspiration. Someone may have communicative skills but lack inspiration, or be inspired but unable to communicate. The best results come from a combination of both.

When we come in at a deeper level, one that we feel ourselves, we do so from our most recent discoveries. Inspirational teaching comes directly from our immediate physical experience. Individual needs are not neglected by targeting the deeper areas for the group as a whole. The experience and understanding provided by our own deep inquiry forms the basis for group work. We can communicate to others as we communicate with ourselves. This is why it helps to *be in it with the group*. Authentic teaching can be a shared experience, flowing in time with time. Inspiration is infectious. An inspired teacher will inspire a deeper group feeling. We might inspire others through our manner and presentation, but group inspiration comes from within each participant. We inspire them to light their own fire; they might be initially inspired by us and then by their own sensations and explorations.

Communication

Communicating deep movement involves the same elements as other work, but the focus is deeper. Practice is physiological, and physiology took care of itself for many years before we applied technique. Sensation has no method as we guide others into places that may be familiar to us, but less so to them. We guide them towards feeling their tissues, bones, articulations and fluid base. We set things up so they can learn from their own experience. Our presence, intuition, voice, language, demonstration and physical contact focus on their potential for an original experience.

Presence

Presence is a form of contact and the foundation of teaching. The depth of your own work deepens your presence in the group. This is picked up by the group before any words are spoken. When you are *there* in yourself, the teaching comes. The deeper and quieter your understanding, the more *there* you will be, without effort or technique. Exercising presence is liberating for the teacher and students. Presence enhances attention and provides the space for authenticity. A natural 'listening to what is' invites the group into a shared space. Group presence puts the group into self-contact. The work begins with presence.

Intuition and Instinct

Intuition is a credible aspect of teaching. *Intuit* may be defined as 'to receive knowledge by direct perception'. *Intuition* is defined in the English Oxford Dictionary as 'the immediate apprehension of an object by the mind without the intervention of any reasoning process'. Intuition can also refer to instinct. *Instinct* relates to an innate impulse or natural tendency, manifesting in acts that appear to be rational but are performed without conscious adaption of means to ends. It also implies an animated force or principle. Instinct arises from the same source as primal movement and could not be more suited to teaching this work. Instinct driving a description or explanation comes from your own body. Your understanding of your own body impels you to guide others into where they might be going or what they might feel.

Go with your instinct; trust it. Trust the group as you open up in their presence and they will be inspired to open more. Teaching may involve a little courage as we expose our deeper selves. Intuition is prolific when we function from impersonality, when we empty from within and expose the inner creature in ourselves. We can show students how *we* are in the work as we loosen our own individuality. We are not imposing our own experience on others but guiding them towards their own deeper discoveries.

Voice

The voice is a powerful tool for touching others. Human sound predates language; the foetus responds to its mother's voice. Human sound is primal, and our voice when used appropriately stirs primal activity. The voice is sound with content. How we speak, our intonations, timbre, texture and tone, what we say, and the timing of the words reach out. The voice holds the group, inspires trust, relaxation, confidence, produces technical understanding and *brings out feeling*. Cultivating all aspects of voice work enables participants to move into and beyond themselves, and gives each member of the group the feeling that you are talking directly to them. The quality of sound and its content draws out each person's creativity. The effects are profound.

The way we describe the spine and its way of moving is a form of touch, as students convert suggestion into feeling. Sound without words can be used when you sense students are being drawn into their rational brain or 'over-thinking' and inhibiting their awareness. Mmmmmm or aaaahhhh, can work well and

put people back into primal mode (like babies). Long pauses between words or sentences work well; for example: 'Come to the end of the exhalation – deeply inside yourself – and – wait – for an inhale to arise – from a deep – unknowable place.'

An unfinished sentence can give an opportunity for students to arrive at their experience while free from your completed suggestion: 'Wait for the pelvis to – and then – '.

Softening, lightening, deepening or just changing tone holds interest, so that you are not monotoning. Ultimately, your voice and how you use it will work for you and for your students. Sometimes the voice and its content is more like a commentary on a current event; it is beyond teaching as the group moves into a collective fluid experience. We are verbally articulating the articular nature of intervertebral activity. Silence will ensue, if and when – .

Deeper

When you are *in it with the group*, they sense your participation and respond by opening their inner creative space and receptivity to deeper and more integrated sensations. We communicate our personal experience to the personal experience of others. Whatever form personal patterns may take, the underlying possibilities remain the same. Because we are not attempting to perfect the *shape* of postures, we can sink beneath the patterns and work from inside out. Someone with less flexibility may access depth as easily as someone with a greater range of movement.

Repetition

Some students may be unable to feel your suggestions. This is the challenge. This is why we should keep going, keep repeating the suggestions and observations, bringing the group back to their deeper potential. Repetition brings the mind back to the relevant sensory appreciation. You cannot mention the exhalation, the pause or the deep spine enough times, sometimes in succession like a mantra. Softening your voice prevents overload. When you shift the focus to another part of the body, keep the attention on primary aspects, reiterate the primary contact points with the ground. When referring to skin or tissues return to central focus and re-establish the relationship between the inner and outer body. If the rhythm is producing fluidity, keep the attention on fluidity.

Organic expression responds to repeating general suggestions such as: 'as you exhale, exhale, as you exhale in the pause', 'be soft, soft, soft', 'as the weight goes down', 'give yourself away', 'wait, wait, wait, for the arrival of the in breath', 'pull yourself together on the out breath, soften on the in breath', and so on.

Changing Position and Reorganising Bones

Organic work invites organic teaching. As bodies deepen and the action 'takes off', the group is drawn into ways of moving that go beyond the frameworks used to 'get things going'. Promoting a deeper feeling involves organising the bones to reduce habitual tissue tension. The possibilities within each basic position should enable spontaneous movement. The skeleton can be rearranged in relation to the ground, and its bones in relation to one another, particularly with regard to the limbs and the spine. You will be familiar with this approach from your own practice.

Suggesting positional variations provide a framework but only as a starting point. Personal exploration should be encouraged. Reorganising positions, varying the angles of the limbs or head, changing position, even slightly, provides a new focus, holds the interest, avoids inertia and gives everyone another route through which to access the spine, pelvis and diaphragm. Changing the angle of limbs and the head can centre bones, deepen breathing, re-establish contact with the ground and remind the group that we are organisms unfolding and unwinding together: Laying the group down following several positions and exploratory movements, and working with the breath, enables them to sense the changes that are

taking place, the additional space, fluidity and articular refinement.

Suggestions should strike an accessible balance between engaging and relaxing: breath work and body work — gathering and opening — skeletal, articular, soft tissue, fluid and spatial possibilities — what we do and how we are.

We are introducing others to their vertebral nature. We can move through our spines as a group, pausing at this or that key vertebra. We can focus on several specific areas in turn as we move through the vertebrae and then bring specific sensations together as one feeling.

Being Touched by the Group

We not only *see* unwanted tension in students, we can feel their tension in our bodies. The group touches our sensory mechanism. An unspoken sense when bodies talk to each other draws us in to how others feel and what they need. You can sense a tense shoulder in your own shoulder or feel another spine in your own spine. As the group opens to its own experience, we immerse with them. We invite them into our experience and enter into theirs. Being in the work yourself, while holding and directing a group, facilitates the appropriate words and their timing. One is within one's own sensory system while simultaneously engaging with others.

Remaining in your neocortical brain to teach, while being fed by your more ancient layers, is an art. You are dividing your mind: one half is in the room and the other half is in yourself. We are juggling between new brain and old brain activity in a teaching situation. This can be very effective but one has to be aware of the possibility of losing oneself and need to keep the focus on the group.

When we are with them in every sense, physiologically, psychologically and emotionally, when we are 'all in it together' and feeling together, the line between teacher and group blurs. Some of the best work and more profound breakthroughs occur in an atmosphere of total harmony between all participants, including the teacher. The group 'field' creates a supportive energy; many people find a deeper place within themselves. If we are teaching organically, and consider group energy and the atmosphere in the room, we create a level playing field, i.e. participants and teacher sharing one field of consciousness. Group consciousness tends to release an energy that is supportive and promotes individual progress. The quality of group consciousness is enhanced when we avoid individual attention unless really necessary. Personal attention, if necessary in this situation, is best conducted without fuss and with a soft voice. Everyone can hear and feel what's going on.

Work in concert with the group, share the experience, but over-reliance on this removes you from individual needs, as a balance always works well.

each student. Within a framework of discovery, *each person is moving in time with their time – their movement of now.* While positional recommendations should be continually acknowledged, the deep flow of involuntary movement is the source of learning. The quality of class work is founded on an uninterrupted inner movement of each person and of the group as a whole. Each participant has their individual rate of emergence, depending upon personal patterns, the depth of their breath and the quality of their gravitation. At the same time, the group finds itself moving and working as a unified organism.

Holding Attention

You can see and feel attention waver as it happens. We know 'when the room begins to lose it'. Stimulation or calming may be required, but with depth work we always return to the common purpose and central focus involving the breath and the feeling of what's happening. Keep the group 'there'; keep bringing the group back to the basic sensations.

Anatomical reference is helpful but easily overdone. Excessive detail has the effect of dulling the senses. It is useful to repeat the essentials that are felt more easily; for example, the shape of the diaphragm, middle of the lumbar curve, the feel of the tail bone and its rhythm, the relationship between vertebrae, shape of the pelvis, length and design of the femur and so on. With a group of teachers you can open up the anatomy, but even then it is easy to overdo it and give an anatomical overload. Give students the map, but maps are the doors to a deeper experience. Anatomical directives keep the attention, but at some point, as the softening and fluid feeling predominates, specific anatomical features blend as a part of one physiological soup, having little, if any, demarcation or delineative margins within the whole.

The skill is to keep people interested, attentive, relaxed and totally involved in their own process. You can teach methods and techniques but nothing satisfies more than acknowledging what is going on *now* for

Demonstrating

It is helpful to show, in yourself or in another, how the body moves from deep within. This demonstrates how the spine, tail, diaphragm, abdominal area, bones and articulations move with the breath in an ancient orchestrated inner dance. You can see primal movement come to the surface. You can highlight another person's movement, or the dance of your own spine.

Feeling the Group

We teach from what we see and from what we feel in our own body-minds. We might sense what others may be feeling but we cannot feel for them. We can, however, set up sensory possibilities.

No two spines are alike, and no two diaphragms have the same tensional qualities. Different people need different things at different times. Original work recognises that beneath the differences we come from the same place within ourselves. We begin *to move in a way that respects individuality yet frees us from it.*

As tension evaporates, our spring-like fluid nature responds. The group feels and looks like an aggregate of ancient creatures, unwinding on a rock, a wild place, a beach, innocently attracted to the dawning of primitive movement, unphased by methods or the intrusion of thought. These concepts give a plausible yet creative setting to the work because we carry their reality in our genetic make-up. They also provide a basis for the imaginative use of language.

Creative Communication

We can't rely on what we did during the previous session. The principle remains the same but language, tempo, group dynamic, sheer mood and an ever-deepening interest lead us into unknown territory. From moment to moment, group work is an immersion into total creativity, for teacher and participants alike. Creature – creation – creativity: our creature created itself in response to its environment. Creative work furthers and refines this response. We recapitulate a time when human form was in creation. As the group reconnects to the earth, breath, spine and primality, the slate is wiped clean, the creature awakens and creativity finds new interpretations. We cannot help but be creative because awakening and emergence are creative phenomena. Creation is present; time is creation. The future might see modifications in form as bony shapes respond to changing life-styles and ways of being. *Refer to the group as primal creatures, unwinding at the dawn of evolution, as embryos growing their spines and limbs, unfolding during the early stages of growth, as creatures opening up to the future.*

Touching

If you teach, you probably touch. Yoga teachers have the potential for delivering, and do deliver, some of the best hands-on work. Many teachers have covered 'adjustments' on training courses and develop them accordingly. Others, through the depth and insight arising from practice, have an affinity with touch as an extension of their personal practice and experience. There are workshops that include the finer aspects of hands-on work, but this is not the place to discuss the pros and cons or details of touching to enhance progress. In any

event, the nature of hands-on work renders it impossible to impart on any in-depth level; it is a practice in itself. How would you encourage a snake to rediscover its primal nature? The following pointers do not include structured techniques, i.e. where and how to touch certain areas, what lies beneath our hands and so on. A manual might do justice to this aspect of our work, which is guided by ever-changing sensation, and at some point beyond the limitations of technique. In terms of facilitating primal movement, a few observations and suggestions might be useful.

The student to be touched is working, and it can be appropriate and easy to facilitate progress and instil a deeper sense of feeling by using one's hands. Make contact from what you see, coupled with your feeling of their body in your own body, e.g. spine-to-spine sensations. We touch on the outside to influence underlying tissue, bones and articulations and the person, who is very much on the inside.

Touching/holding should facilitate depth of expression. An effective way forward is to *bring parts of the body towards each other.* This releases the large muscles, gives back to the spine and invites depth sense to proliferate into spontaneous movement. The long bones fulfil this requirement. Holding the limbs and feeding them back to the centre releases and activates the spine. This involves finding suitable angles for a thigh or upper arm bone, and changing the angle to appeal to a different level of the spine. Encouraging an approximation of the shoulder blades can be effective in releasing the thoracic spine.

The same approach can be used for shoulder or pelvic releases and stimulation, head holding, rib involvement and vertebral inclusion. The spine can be accessed by direct contact or through the agency of the limbs. This work invites subtlety and sensitivity. There is no ambition on the part of the teacher, simply a facilitation of something that wants to happen or is happening.

The 'sucking back and up' as the abdominal muscles follow the diaphragm can be facilitated by a hand on the belly. Sometimes a hand on heel, or elbow, hip, angle of the ribs, or shoulder, can stimulate sensory depth. The body can respond to the slightest and lightest contact.

Facilitating through touch acknowledges personal patterns as well as the expression common to all. We are not adjusting people into positions but working within the framework of a given attitude.

We engage in moment-to-moment contact with another organism. The sensations arising from our contact travels through our tissues and spine into awareness. Any objective is coloured by feeling. We impart awareness, depth and space while encouraging interconnectivity and rhythm. The mechanical aspects of facilitation are the same as those in personal practice and we should be aware that stretching a body inhibits its rhythmic expression. Facilitation is a practice. There are times when a group moves so freely and creatively that touching is an interference. The rhythm is inherent; it enables itself.

Working with Teachers

You may have teachers or trainee teachers in a group who appreciate anatomical references and philosophical insights from a renewed and alternative perspective. One may have teachers and non-teachers in the same group. Non-teachers always benefit from aspects directed at teachers. Everyone is touched by a common profundity. A general approach may prevail because depth work sinks beneath the *idea of teaching*. Individuals will take and use what they need at the time. We cannot teach others to teach, and although a structure or 'course' might suit, we can only find the art of teaching in ourselves, in the same way that we can only find the art of practice in ourselves. Practice and teaching spring from the same source. There are some excellent teachers who have never attended teacher training courses, but have had some inspiring teachers. On the other hand, if someone finds the right course it can only help. The important thing is not to get lost in the course. If you are teaching, you know how to teach; you might simply be changing the focus.

Channelling

The channelling experience is common. It can feel as if we channel an intelligence, as if something or someone comes through us. We are aware of it and so is the group. We speak and act in a way that is beyond our personality and ego. These experiences may come from beneath what we know, an older and wiser voice emerging from the primal centres into consciousness as we open up our body-minds to the group. Speech may be particularly slow, every word measured and relevant, as the frontal brain opens up to a deeper energy. The group senses this 'otherness' and responds by tapping more deeply into their origins.

You will Know

Your body will sense what is happening in the group. You will know how, where, and when to use your voice, language and touch and when to be silent. You will know how to bring out original activity in others. As movement unfolds, you will know when to organise bones, return to the breath, address fluidity, provide anatomical reference, or pause to highlight 'how we are' by acknowledging the effects of where we have been and where we might be going. You will know when to bring in anatomical, philosophical or anecdotal aspects related to the work.

You will know it through the symbiotic relationship in the room, between you and the group and between group members. You will know when to act and when to stand back. But you cannot know in advance; you cannot plan where and when to intercede. This unknown and unplanned element of teaching produces the best results.

Working with new students takes particular patience when introducing something a little different. 'I can't feel it' comes up time and again. Many people need time to reawaken their sensory system on a deeper level. There is no time frame; it may take hours or weeks depending on the student, but every session is progressive. A whole group of new students is obviously more challenging than having one or two new participants in a regular group. There is no special formula other than to keep going, with the understanding that the 'organism knows' and will respond at some point. The energy of those who have been with you for some time will carry the newcomers to some extent.

Working deeply with several positions followed by insightful, but short, discussion is an interesting way of working. If you consider the acknowledgement of 'how we are' as an integral aspect of what we do, students find this approach useful and affirming. If you are so inclined, it can be useful to open up the nature of the work, philosophically, anatomically, personally and in terms of the bigger picture. This cannot be planned but comes through inspired spontaneity. We can return to the 'exercises' at any point.

Common sense is a *sense*. We sense with it and act on what we sense. We cannot teach common sense – it is implicit in our nature although perhaps more in some than others – but it is there. Technique and enthusiasm can easily override common sense. Common inherency responds most readily to an approach founded on common sense. We find even more common sense as we deepen our own practice and our conditioning lifts.

Life Experience and Common Sense

At any one time we may be facilitators, mentors, mechanics, anatomists, therapists and sometimes entertainers. Teaching others combines any mix of anatomy, technique, philosophy, references to behaviour or love, sometimes during the same moments, plus the essential, unavoidable presence of our own *life experience*. Without imposing in any way, our personal history, ups and downs, our view of life, tempered by all we have learnt, aspects of our individual conditioning, within the grand scheme of things, provide the bedrock upon which all other aspects of teaching rests. Insight is based on personal experience of the past blending with the experience of being present. Insight is the consequence of the movement of the past flowing through now into next. We simply let it through, leaving the rest to 'common sense'.

Where does common sense come from? If we need anything at all as teachers, it is common sense. Common sense enables us to pick up what is needed at any given moment and rise to the occasion.

Symbiosis

As teachers, we draw people together for the common purpose of deepening their experience, and in so doing move beyond and beneath habitual patterns. Symbiosis played a major role in our evolution. Cooperation between organisms underpins our continuance as a species. We are *symbiotes* with work in progress, mutually engaged in relaxing egos, dissolving personalities and coming together in an ancient rhythm common to all. The deeper we go, the closer we feel, as personal patterns float to the periphery of awareness. Love emerges and behaviour changes as we bathe together in the light of a less conditioned, more refined way of being. If this can in some way make a difference within our sphere of influence, we are making a contribution to the general state of play. In coming together and 'working in' as opposed to 'working out', we provide an opportunity for ourselves and for those with us, to realise a more profound, stronger and potentially enlightened way of being.

References

Alexander, Matthias F 1932 (1985) *The use of the self.* London: Victor Gollancz.

Baba Ram Dass 1977 *Grist for the mill.* New York: Harperone.

Baker, Elsworth F 1967 *Man in the trap.* New York: MacMillan Publishing.

Barks, Coleman 1997 *The essential Rumi.* New Jersey: Castle Books, Harper Collins.

Buzzell, Keith 1970 *The philsiological basis of osteopathic medicine.* New York: Insight Publishing, Ch. 4, 72.

Conrad, Emilie 2007 *Life on land.* Berkeley: CA: North Atlantic Books.

Damasio, Antonio 1999 *The feeling of what happens.* London: Random House.

Desikachar, TKV 1982 *The yoga of T. Krishnamacharya.* Madras: The Krisnamachrya Yoga Mandiram.

Ellis, George FR 2008 *The flow of time.* University of Cape Town SA: Mathematics Department.

England, Marjorie A 1983 *A colour atlas of life before birth.* UK: Woolfe Medical Publications.

Feldenkrais, Moshe 2010 Embodied wisdom. In: **Elizabeth Beringer,** ed. *The collected papers of Moshe Feldenkrais.* Berkeley: North Atlantic Books.

Feldenkrais, Moshe 2005 *Body and mature behaviour.* Berkeley: North Atlantic Books.

Feldenkrais, Moshe 1949 *Body and mature behavior: a study of anxiety, sex, gravitation and learning.* London: **Routledge and Kegan Paul,** New York: International Universities Press.

Feldenkrais, Moshe 1995 Breath, bone and gesture. In: **Don Hanlon Johnson,** ed. *The illusive obvious.* Capitola: Meta Publications.

Feuerstein, Georg 2003 *The deeper dimension of yoga.* Boston: Shambala Publications.

Feuerstein, Georg 1997 *Lucid waking.* Rochester, Vermont: Inner Traditions International.

Freud, Sigmund 1930 *Civilisation and its discontents,* 8th impression. London: Hogarth Press.

Freud, Sigmund. 1927 *Ego and the id.* revised edn, 1962. London: Hogarth Press and Institute of Phychoanalysis.

Fromme, Erich 1976 *To have or to be.* New York: Harper Row, 1978 London: Jonathan Cape.

Funderburk, James 1977 *Science studies yoga.* USA: Himalayan Institute of Yoga Science and Philosophy of USA.

Gray 1989 *Gray's anatomy,* 37th edn. Edinburgh: Churchill Livingstone.

Gebser, Jean 1945 *The ever present origin.* Columbus: University Press.

Gracovetsky, Serge 1989 *The spinal engine.* New York: Springer-Verlag.

Hamilton, David R 2010 *Why kindness is good for you.* London: Hay House.

Hanson, Rick 2009 *Buddha's brain.* Oakland: New Harbinger Publications.

Hartranft, Chip 2003 *The yoga sutra of Patanjali.* Boston: Shambala Publications.

Hawking, Stephen 1988 *A brief history of time.* London: Bantam Press.

Horney, Karen 1937 *The neurotic personality of our time.* New York: W. W. Norton.

Husserl in Gebser Jean 1949 *The ever present origin.* Columbus, OH: Ohio University Press.

Iyengar, BKS 1987 *Iyengar his life and work,* 2nd edn. New Delhi: **SK Jane** for CBS Publishers.

Juhan, Deane 1987 *Job's body.* New York: Station Hill Press.

Korr, Irvin M 1951 *The collected papers of Irvin Korr*, 4th printing 1993. Indianapolis: American Academy of Osteopathy.

Krishnamurti, J 1954 *The first and last freedom*. New York: Harper Collins.

Krisnamurti, J 1969 *Freedom from the known*. New York: Harper Collins.

Laing, RD 1983 *The voice of experience*. New York: Random House.

Laing, RD 1960 *The divided self*. London: Penguin Classics 2010.

Langevin, Helene, Huijing, Peter 2009 *Communicating about fascia*. International Journal of Therapeutic Massage and Bodywork 2(4):3–8.

Lewis, Thomas, Amini, Fari, Lannon, Richard 2000 *The general theory of love*. New York: Vintage Books, Random House.

Lipton, Bruce 2005 *The biology of belief*. New York: Hay House.

Littlejohn, John Martin 1898 *Principles and practice of osteopathy*. Kirksville: Journal Printing Company.

Lowen, Alexander 1958 *The language of the body*. Hinesburg: The Alexander Lowen Foundation.

Manaka, Yoshio 1995 *Chasing the Dragon's Tail*. Boulder: Paradigm Publishers.

McLynn, Frank 1996 *A biography, Carl Gustav Jung*. London: Transworld Publishers.

McTaggart, Lynn 2001 *The field*. New York: Harper Collins.

Montague, Ashley 1971 *Touching, the human significance of the skin*. New York: Harper Row.

Odent, Michel 1999 *The scientification of love*. London: Free Association Books Ltd.

Osho 1996 *The birth of being*. New York: Osho International Foundation.

Oschman, James 2000 *Energy medicine, the scientific basis*. Philadelphia: Elsevier.

Oxford English Dictionary 1977 Oxford: Oxford University Press.

Postgraduate Institute of Osteopathic Medicine and Surgery 1970 *The physiological basis of osteopathic medicine*; adapted from the symposium presented October 7, 1967. New York: Insight.

Reich, Wilhelm 1942 *Function of the orgasms*, 1975 edn. New York: Pocket Books.

Reich, Wilhelm 1933 *Character analysis*. New York: Farrar, Straus and Giroux.

Rolf, Ida 1977 *Rolfing, the integration of human structures*. New York: Harper Row.

Staubesand, J, Li, Y 1996 In: Chaitow, Leon *Naturopathic physical medicine: theory and practice for manual therapists*. Edinburgh: Elsevier.

Schleip, Robert 2012 *Fascia as a sensory organ*. In: *The Tensional Network of the Human Body: The science and clinical applications in manual and movement therapy*. Edinburgh: Elsevier.

Schwenk, Theodor 1962 *Sensitive chaos*, revised Translation 1996. London: Rudolph Steiner.

Simmel in Gebser 1945 *The ever present origin*. Columbus: Ohio University Press.

Still, Andrew Taylor 1902 *The philosophy and mechanical principles of osteopathy* 1986 edn. Kirksville: Osteopathic Enterprise.

Sweigard, Lulu 1974 *Human movement potential, its ideokinetic facilitation*. New York: Harper Row.

Todd, Mabel 1937 *The thinking body*. Hightstown, NJ: Princeton Book Company, A Dance Horizon Book.

Todd, Mabel 1953 *The hidden you*. Brooklyn: Dance Horizons.

Tortora, Gerard J, Anagnostakos, Nicholas P 1990 *Principles of anatomy and physiology*, 6th edn. New York: Harper Row.

Upledger, John E, Vredevoogd, John D 1983 *Craniosacral therapy*. Seattle: Eastland Press.

van der Wal, Jaap 2012 **Proprioception. In:** *The Tensional Network of the Human Body: The science and clinical applications in manual and movement.* **Edinburgh: Elsevier Ltd.**

van der Wal, Jaap 2003 *Speech of the embryo*. Betty Reiniers editor. London: Craniosacral Therapy Educational Trust.

Index